Praise for *The 100-Year Lifestyle*

"As a soon to be centenarian 'well' on my way to the 100 mark, I applaud the guidelines set forth in Dr. Plasker's book, *The 100-Year Lifestyle.*"

—Jack LaLanne

"Dr. Plasker has committed many years to developing health and wellness programs for communities around the country. His book reflects this same commitment and will help you improve the quality of your life."

—Stedman Graham, founder of Athletes Against Drugs

"Dr. Plasker's innovative 100-Year Lifestyle Fitness Assessment on getting your ESS in shape—your endurance, strength, and structure—will help you add years to your life and quality of life to your years."

—Scott Goudeseune, president, American Council on Exercise

"Dr. Plasker's care and 100-Year Lifestyle concepts have helped me greatly improve my competitiveness and I am certain will ultimately extend my athletic career. I have always put a great deal of stress on my spine and skeletal structure, especially while training for the world record modified bench press, and with the help of Dr. Plasker's care I was able to set the world record of 360 pounds in March of 2004. You need this in your life!"

—Kyle Maynard, world record holder
and bestselling author of *No Excuses*

"Dr. Plasker reveals the time-tested principles to living your best life in this easy-to-read guide that makes living well a reality for all. Discover how to dramatically increase both the quality and the quantity of your years. Read this book as if your life actually depends on it, because it does."

—Bob Hoffman D.C., CEO of the Masters Circle and coauthor
of *Discover Wellness: How Staying Healthy Can Make You Rich*

"With Dr. Eric Plasker to guide the way, there's no reason to dread getting older. His advice can help all of us enjoy a century full of life, health, energy, and passion. His book—packed with incredible, life-enhancing principles and advice—shows once more why Dr. Plasker is considered one of the nation's foremost health and wellness experts."

—Terry A. Rondberg, D.C., president, World Chiropractic Alliance

Praise for *The 100-Year Lifestyle*

"Dr. Plasker's principles make living to 100 exciting, rather than frightening. You will benefit from these life changing health, relationship, and financial principles today, tomorrow, and every day for the rest of your life."

—Ivan Misner, Ph.D., founder of BNI
and *New York Times* bestselling author

"Dr. Plasker's *100-Year Lifestyle* will take you from Good to Great to Exceptional! I have been involved in the wellness industry for over 29 years and have never met a more suited, devoted, intelligent, caring, and driven person than Dr. Plasker. Read, Live, and Sleep with this book; it has the power to enhance your life. With his guidance you will reach a happy and healthy 100."

—Doug Caporrino, international speaker
and trainer to the stars

"Dr. Plasker has created the opportunity for people to live the health of their dreams at every age. This book is fun to read, very practical, and easy to follow. I really appreciate the reflective points and self-responsibility it promotes. Well done. Again, an ounce of prevention is worth a pound of cure."

—Dr. Liz Anderson-Peacock,
CEO, Girls, Gals and Gurus Inc.,
a healthy lifestyle company for women

In *The 100-Year Lifestyle,* Dr. Plasker addresses a marvelous question that our over-stressed society must think about, 'What if I were to live to 100?' As this book points out, the implications are huge. In the chaotic world of wellness, this book stands out as unique, powerful, and immensely practical . . . not to mention, it is a lot of fun. Read this and learn to live well, to 100 and beyond."

—Patrick Gentempo, Jr., D.C., CEO, Creating Wellness, Inc.

The 100 Year Lifestyle™

DR. ERIC PLASKER'S BREAKTHROUGH SOLUTION FOR LIVING YOUR BEST LIFE—EVERY DAY OF YOUR LIFE!

ERIC PLASKER, D.C., Internationally Acclaimed Wellness Expert

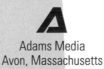

Adams Media
Avon, Massachusetts

Published by
Adams Media, an F+W Publications Company
57 Littlefield Street, Avon, MA 02322. U.S.A.
www.adamsmedia.com

ISBN 10: 1-59869-093-0
ISBN 13: 978-1-59869-093-4

Printed in the United States of America.

J I H G F E D C B A

Library of Congress Cataloging-in-Publication Data
Plasker, Eric.
The 100-year lifestyle / Eric Plasker.
p.   cm.
ISBN-13: 978-1-59869-093-4 (hardcover)
ISBN-10: 1-59869-093-0 (hardcover)
1. Longevity—Popular works. 2. Aging—Prevention—Popular works.
3. Health—Popular works. I. Title. II. Title: One hundred year lifestyle.
RA776.75.P53 2007
613.2—dc22
2006100751

This publication is designed to provide accurate and authoritative information with regard to the subject matter covered. It is sold with the understanding that the publisher is not engaged in rendering legal, accounting, or other professional advice. If legal advice or other expert assistance is required, the services of a competent professional person should be sought.
—From a *Declaration of Principles* jointly adopted by a Committee of the American Bar Association and a Committee of Publishers and Associations

Many of the designations used by manufacturers and sellers to distinguish their product are claimed as trademarks. Where those designations appear in this book and Adams Media was aware of a trademark claim, the designations have been printed with initial capital letters.

The 100-Year Lifestyle is intended as a reference volume only, not as a medical manual. In light of the complex, individual, and specific nature of heath problems, this book is not intended to replace professional medical advice. The ideas, procedures, and suggestions in this book are intended to supplement, not replace, the advice of a trained medical professional. Consult your physician before adopting the suggestions in this book. The author and publisher disclaim any liability arising directly or indirectly from the use of this book.

This book is available at quantity discounts for bulk purchases.
For information, please call 1-800-289-0963.

CONTENTS

ACKNOWLEDGMENTS

The 100-Year Lifestyle comes from both my inborn desire to help people, and a lifetime of experiences and relationships. I am thankful to all of the people who have contributed to my journey.

I am thankful that God has blessed me with the talents and abilities to help so many people and make a difference.

I'd like to wish my grandfather, Hyman Sperling, a happy 100th birthday. Congratulations on becoming a centenarian.

Lisa, my wife of eighteen years, thank you for standing by me, as well as for being my partner in life and an incredible mother to our children. I love you.

To my children, Jacob, Emily and Cory, I could never be more proud of you. Continue to search for your niche in the world and apply yourself to the things that you love. Remember to take care of yourselves and take care of each other. I love you all and I love being your dad.

My mom and dad are great parents and have given me so much over the years. Mom, thank you for passing your passion to me of wanting to help people reach their full potential. Dad, I wish you could read this book. You would be proud. Since you fell ill, my sense of urgency to complete this work has been accelerated. You have been such a strong, positive force in my life. I miss you very much.

My brothers, Dr. Jordan and Dr. Noel Plasker, are my best friends. You guys are an incredible source of strength for me. Seeing our families love each other so much means the world to me.

To my mother and father in-law, Herb and Joanne Singer, thank you for embracing me into your family and loving my children.

I have been blessed with a huge family of cousins—some of my best friends in the world. There is no way to mention them all.

I have been blessed with so many great mentors and coaches over the years. From Ed Huber to Chuck Scarpula and Tony Amarillo, your leadership started me on the right track.

In my professional life, my mentors in chiropractic have been extraordinary. Dr. Ernie Landi, thank you for my first adjustment and for telling me the story. Drs. Alex, Doug, and Jon Cox, thank you for your expertise and for teaching me to be an excellent doctor. Dr. Guy Reikeman, thank you for connecting me to the big idea and inspiring me to make a difference. Dr. Joseph Flesia, you have impacted me more than anyone in my professional life. Your teachings and your memory inspire me every day.

My team at The Family Practice has given me incredible support. Dr. Cheryl Langley, Dr. Carmelo Caratozzolo, Dr. Russ Pavkov, Dr. Gary Brodeur, Dr. Tina Theriot, Dr. Bart Rzepa, Dr. Craig Pruitt, Dr. Miguel Cruz, Phyllis Frase, Dr. Scott Stachelek, and Dr. Terry Harmon, let's continue to help as many people as possible reach their full potential.

Thank you to all of my thousands of patients over the years who taught me about health and healing, human potential, hope and possibility. Your belief in me nurtured the seeds of this book and made me realize the importance of taking a stand for people.

Thank you to my good friends and mentors over the years including Dr. Fabrizio Mancini, Mark Victor Hansen, Jack Canfield, Barbara De Angelis, Dan Sullivan, Dr. Patrick Gentempo, Doug Caporrino, Dr. Carol Ann Malilia, Dr. Bob Hoffman, Dr. Sid Williams, Dr. Gerald Clum, Dr. Ari Diskin, Dr. Glenn Maginess, and Stedman Graham to name a few.

I would like to thank my entire book team who helped give birth to this important work. To Robyn and Willy Spizman, thanks for that first thirty-minute meeting that turned into two and a half hours, then two and a half years, and a book that will impact a lot of lives. Thanks to my writer, Jill Westfall, for your thoroughness, dedication, creativity and persistence with this project. You are a true professional. Also, thanks to Jenifer Wadsworth for helping me to kick this project into existence.

To Paula, Gary, Karen, Beth, Meredith, and everyone else at Adams Media, thank you for believing in me, this book, and putting all your creativity and energy behind it. Let's enjoy a sensational century.

THE 100-YEAR LIFESTYLE ASSESSMENT
TAKE THE LEAP!

Are you living the 100-Year Lifestyle? Find out by honestly answering the following questions about your current life.

NEVER   **ALWAYS**

I am excited about the possibility of living to 100

1	2	3	4	5

I have many goals that I would like to achieve over my extended life

1	2	3	4	5

I am willing to make changes to improve my quality of life as I age

1	2	3	4	5

I have youthful energy in spite of my age

1	2	3	4	5

I enjoy a full night of restful sleep and feel energized each morning

1	2	3	4	5

I can consciously shift my energy whenever I want to

1	2	3	4	5

I am aware of the diseases in my family history

1	2	3	4	5

I live a lifestyle that counteracts the diseases in my family history

1	2	3	4	5

I am motivated by quality of life health goals rather than crisis management

1	2	3	4	5

I feel good about my current health condition

1	2	3	4	5

I exercise 4 to 5 times a week and am getting the results I want from my fitness routine

1	2	3	4	5

I eat healthy foods and supplement my diet

1	2	3	4	5

NEVER   **ALWAYS**

I visit health care providers proactively to stay healthy and avoid unnecessary health problems

1	2	3	4	5

I live in a peaceful, stress-free home environment

1	2	3	4	5

I work in an environment that nurtures my talents and where I feel appreciated

1	2	3	4	5

My home and work environment reflect my inner feelings and voice

1	2	3	4	5

I support myself through choices that I know are good for me

1	2	3	4	5

I actively seek out opportunities and enjoy learning new things

1	2	3	4	5

I am surrounded by supportive relationships at home and at work

1	2	3	4	5

I have achieved the balance I am looking for

1	2	3	4	5

I am able to separate work time from play time

1	2	3	4	5

I have a clear picture of how I want to use my time during my extended life

1	2	3	4	5

My current financial path can sustain me until I reach 100

1	2	3	4	5

I am passionate about work and the way I earn money

1	2	3	4	5

I am living within my means and saving money regularly

1	2	3	4	5

I feel like my life has purpose and I am making a difference

1	2	3	4	5

I am actively involved in my community

1	2	3	4	5

I have a mentor and I use my leadership skills to mentor others

1	2	3	4	5

Add all the circled numbers. This is your total score.

❏ If your score was 0 to 35:

Slam on the Brakes and Change Your Life

You are either in denial, at the end of your rope, or just don't care. At the rate you are going both your mind and your body are headed for trouble. You are taking years off your life and will be a financial burden to your children or society. It's not too late to turn things around. Keep reading and embrace the Three Life-Changing Principles of the 100-Year Lifestyle to make the remaining years of your life the best. Take the Lifestyle Leap and pay close attention to the Three Life-Changing Principles in Chapter 2!

❏ If your score was 36 to 70:

Stop Killing Yourself Slowly

At the rate you are going you are headed for a deteriorating and depressing extended life. You have no vision, poor habits, and lack a sense of purpose. You are using crisis as the motivation to take action on the habits that you know are good for you, rather than embracing the quality of life you deserve. Stop compromising yourself. You can simply, steadily, and easily make 100-Year Lifestyle changes to enjoy your longevity with the health, passion, and meaning to make it all worthwhile. Take the Lifestyle Leap and enjoy the youthful energy and enthusiasm that you will learn about in Chapters 3 and 4!

❏ If your score was 71 to 105:

Get Ready to Go from Good to Great

You are probably on a roller coaster filled with ups and downs. You are enjoying your life, but you are out of balance with swings that go too far to the extreme. Some things are working well for you, while other areas of your life are out of control. Address the areas of the 100-Year Lifestyle that will impact your life the most and you will find that your life gets easier, your results go up, and you start having a lot more fun. You will add better health, financial security, peace of mind, and purpose to an already solid foundation. Take the Lifestyle Leap and discover how to attract new friends, find new passions, and achieve the balance you are looking for by embracing the ideas in Chapters 14, 15, 16 and 17!

❏ If your score was 106-140:

Enjoy a Sensational Century

You are on your way. You are living your dreams while you plan for the future, both at the same time. You enjoy your work and feel like you can do it forever. The good news is that by following this plan, it won't be something you have to do, but something you can choose to do if you want to. You are in good health, you have goals to achieve, and a world of opportunity ahead of you. Embracing the 100-Year Lifestyle will ensure that you enjoy your legacy while you are alive, enjoy youthful energy and passion, and make the most of this precious gift called your life. Take the Lifestyle Leap by refining your life vision, having more fun than ever, and making your life matter by adopting the concepts in Chapters 17, 19 and 20!

INTRODUCTION

If you knew you'd live to 100, how would you change your life? One of the world's most famous centenarians, George Burns, summed it up well when he joked that had he known he was going to live to be 100, he would have taken better care of himself. Never has a punch line more profoundly put the aging process in the proper perspective! Let this irony open the doorway to smart choices that can support you in every way as your genealogy edges you toward the increasing probability that you will live to 100 or longer!

As a dedicated wellness expert, health care consultant, columnist, lecturer, and chiropractor, I have been a catalyst in helping people of all ages maximize the quality and quantity of their lives. They've done it by practicing the change principles I've developed over the past two decades of researching and probing the depths of human potential. Coined a "Change Master" by my colleagues and patients, it's my mission to give you life-enhancing information that generates real transformation in your level of health, prosperity, and happiness.

The truth is staggering. Anyone who is 40 years of age today could live to be 100 years old and their grandchildren could live even longer than that. While this information is exciting to me and to many of my clients, I am taken aback by the large number of people who express a reluctance to ride this road for fear they'll outlive their assets, experience declining health, or be a burden to their family. Unwilling to compromise on my own quality of life as I age, I dedicated my career to teaching audiences around the world how to change their lives and embrace this new lease on longevity and minimize any of its ill effects.

The truth is your body has the hardware to live to 100 years and beyond. Understanding and accepting this genetic opportunity will help you express your unlimited life potential. The 100-Year Lifestyle strategies you uncover in this book will not only help you embrace an extended life span, but teach you how to live life to the fullest and live your best possible legacy while you are alive, rather than just leave it after you are gone.

How will you accept this gift of extra time? Will it be with gratitude or reluctance and more importantly, how will this gift inspire you to change your career, family relationships, and life priorities? Together, we will uncover the anatomy of your extended life span as well as the health, energy, and riches that can be yours as a result of this gift.

If you're going to live to 100 anyway, why not make it a sensational century? Choice and change will fuel your future. Choose to change the way you view, plan, manage, and live your life. Put these change principles into place and maximize your health, wealth, and professional and personal relationships. Create a signature life plan that will prepare you physically, financially, and emotionally to live a joyous life no matter what your age every step of the way. The 100-Year Lifestyle will give you the knowledge and tools for living an incredible life every day of your life for 100 years and beyond.

Meet you there!

Dr. Eric Plasker
Founder of The Family Practice, Inc., and LCfE, LLC

PART 1

Welcome
to the
100-Year
Lifestyle

*If I knew I was going
to live this long,
I would have . . .*

CHAPTER 1
TELL ME SOMETHING I DON'T KNOW

Welcome to the 100-Year Lifestyle. I'll bet this isn't the first book you've purchased hoping to improve the quality of your life. In fact, our world is filled with so much information on the Internet and in the book stores that you may even think you already know all there is to know about building a life of lasting health, wealth, and meaningful relationships. "Tell me something I don't know," you say. But, there's a reason why you bought this book. Could it be that your life is at a crossroads? Maybe you're feeling younger than ever regardless of your age and you want to maximize the opportunities that lie ahead of you. Or maybe you're feeling older than you should and you're ready to rediscover your youthful energy and passion for life. Is it possible that up until now, the messages you've received haven't been meaningful enough to get you to take action? Has changing just seemed like more trouble than it's worth?

Now, let me tell you something you may not know. Change is easy; it's thinking about change that is hard. When you finally have the realization that your parents and grandparents' generation is living nearly twice as long as scientists thought they would, and you probably will too, what will you do about it? Will this be the catalyst for you to make the changes you know you need to make to ensure the quality of life you want and deserve? Will you start taking better care of yourself physically, mentally, socially, and financially? Are you ready to get excited about the rest of your life?

In this book, you are going to find a blueprint for living to 100 years—and beyond. The focus is on maximizing the

quality of your life—and your longevity—by helping you to identify and optimize your own unique genetic potential. It's a fascinating journey and I'm honored to accompany you through it.

Along the way, you will embrace some exciting new concepts
and realities about age and longevity that are life changing. For
example, like it or not, the fact is that our grandparents' generation is living nearly twice as long as scientists thought they
would. They were unprepared for this good fortune and many
have paid the price for it. They didn't think that they would need
their health, finances, or relationships to sustain them for so long
and as a result, they haven't. *For this reason, very few of us regard old
age as something positive.*

You are about to begin seeing things a different way. You'll
even meet 90-year-olds and centenarians, who are already living
the 100-Year Lifestyle today, such as Henry Rohlfs of Short Hills,
New Jersey, who celebrated his ninetieth birthday by taking a
ride in a hot air balloon over Luxor, Egypt. I wonder what kind
of adventures you will choose to make the most of all the decades
that you have left.

You will discover in this book that managing your health
is a lot like managing your money. Good intentions are not
enough—you must back them up with actions. This is so important because if the experts are right and the current aging trends
continue, you'll probably end up living much longer than you
ever imagined.

> **Living the 100-Year Lifestyle** Our longest-lived centenarian is
> Madame Jeanne Calment, who died at the age of 122.

There is tremendous opportunity in the 100-Year Lifestyle,
which will be revealed to you. By planning for your own longevity, you are opening the door to the opportunity of not only "first"
and "second" acts, but "third" and "fourth" acts as well. You are
opening the door to an abundance of new beginnings, knowing
that there is time to accomplish every goal you've ever dreamed
of. You'll substitute refinement for retirement as you maintain a

▶ THE 100-YEAR LIFESTYLE DEFINED

WHAT IT IS . . .

» Living a healthy, passionate, prosperous life, every day of your life, for 100 years and beyond
» Great relationships with multiple generations and multiple circles of people
» Lifelong learning, activity, and adventure
» Financial freedom, abundance, and independence
» The perfect balance of exploration, play time, and fun combined with meaningful work
» Maximizing your genetic capabilities and making the most of your time, energy, and talents
» Keeping your original body parts functioning at full capacity
» Stimulating your mind to keep it sharp
» Accepting challenges, embracing change, and adapting to the unexpected
» Balancing the need for immediate gratification and a secure future
» Knowing and trusting yourself
» Yours to customize

WHAT IT IS NOT . . .

» Rotting away as a human preservative in a nursing home
» Abusing your body, masking symptoms with drugs, and then continuing to abuse yourself until one organ after the other has to be removed or replaced
» All work and no play
» Abusive relationships or isolation
» Financial survival for 35 years and then barely squeaking by on Social Security and Medicare
» Insignificant retirement where you become a meaningless number in a long line of an outdated system
» Wearing out your body in the first 50 years and then suffering the consequences during the second 50 years
» Accumulating wealth in the first 50 years and destroying relationships along the way, leaving you nobody to share it with
» Creating wealth at the price of your health
» Denying yourself the good things in life

sense of productivity, purpose, and passion for life—throughout your entire lifetime.

Understand that life expectancy and life span are two different things. Prior to the twentieth century, life expectancy was about half of what it is today, but the life span was not that different. Many people have been documented as living beyond 90 as far back as the sixteenth century.

What is happening today is that more and more people are reaching the ends of their natural life spans. This is great news, but only when you have planned for it. What you want is a good quality of life—throughout your life. And what you will see in this book is that actions leading to an abundant 100-Year Lifestyle will also optimize the quality of your life today.

It's a fact that centenarians—people who are living to 100 or more—are one of the fastest-growing age groups in the United States and many other industrialized nations around the world. There are now over 50,000 centenarians living in this country. If you are a baby boomer, you'll join the nearly 400 million people around the world who will be 100 years of age or older by 2050 and the estimated 2 million centenarians in the United States alone. Are you ready for this incredible opportunity? Will you enjoy the quality of life that you deserve along the way?

I've spent the last two decades asking thousands of patients and seminar attendees one powerful question, "If you knew you'd live to 100, how would you change your life?" To my surprise, many of them express no desire to live that long. They worry that they will run out of money. They worry they will end up isolated and alone. They don't want to be a cripple or a burden to their family and friends.

So, how do you plan to approach this potential milestone? Will you keep overworking and under-exercising? Will you eat more than you should and be less fulfilled than you could be? Or will you make the most of your journey along the way?

Will knowing that you have the ability to live a century or more lend urgency to your desire to change the way you approach your own aging? A lot of it depends on how you respond to what you think you already know.

Throughout this book, I will give you opportunities to take action on our discussions through Live Long and Strong exercises. Take the action step and get involved in the process to customize your own 100-Year Lifestyle. No one else can live it for you.

CRISIS MOTIVATION VERSUS QUALITY-OF-LIFE MOTIVATION

We live in a society where crisis motivates us to change. It takes a heart attack to get many people to stop smoking, or to eat healthy. When we can't fit into our clothes anymore, we decide to cut calories or to start exercising. It's a paradoxical health approach where

▶ LIVE LONG AND STRONG EXERCISE

If you knew you were going to live to 100, how would you change your life? List the immediate changes that you know deep down in your heart that you need to make:

1. _____
2. _____
3. _____
4. _____
5. _____

What are the long-term and lasting changes you would make?

1. _____
2. _____
3. _____
4. _____
5. _____

illness inspires us to be well. It's one that may leave you punching the nurse call button instead of enjoying the active, healthy life you deserve.

About ten years ago, a 98-year-old man walked into my practice. His name was Max, and he was miserable. He shuffled in with a bent back and arthritic fingers. It hurt just to look at him. Unable to stand upright, Max told me he couldn't bear the pain much longer and he was ready to do whatever it took to improve his quality of life.

After nearly a year of care, Max's discomfort began to subside. His flexibility and mobility slowly began to improve. His crisis appeared over, and Max stopped coming in. For months, my staff made attempts to re-engage him in his wellness adjustment plan, but Max was nowhere to be found. We couldn't contact him by phone, and there were no family members that we could contact. The letters we mailed went unanswered. Eventually, we gave up.

A year later, I was surprised to find Max standing in my doorway. As I got closer to him, I could see that he was weak and tired. He looked like a man who was ready to pass. Within seconds, he collapsed on the counter in my reception room and died. Sadness and shock spread through my staff as the ambulance drove him away. There was nobody to call and no family to console. I understood then why Max had come to my office. He had come there because he had no other place to go.

Max had approached the 100-year mark with no money, no physical strength, no energy, and no loving connections to sustain him. On the surface, it seemed like there was nothing left of Max. But the truth is, he left something huge behind for me.

It was a question mark so large that I could not ignore it. The question was, "If Max had known he was going to live to 100, how would he have changed his life when he was 40, 50, or 60 years old?" Would he have put his health, wealth, and relationships back into balance before the crisis occurred?

You and I both know there is a better way. Living into "old age" doesn't mean outliving your resources, relationships, or joy. In fact, you'll find many older Americans working out at the YMCA, dancing at parties, and traveling the globe. Just look at Jack La-Lanne. This Godfather of Fitness is changing more lives than ever in his nineties. Also in his mid nineties now, Art Linkletter just published a great new book with Mark Victor Hansen called *How to Make the Rest of Your Life the Best of Your Life*. Pianist Arthur Rubinstein still dazzles audiences at 88, and Emma Grady celebrated her 100th birthday by throwing out the first pitch at an Arizona Diamondbacks baseball game. They let their love for life—and desire to be healthy—motivate their choices. They have not let crisis be a catalyst for maintaining their health and vitality.

The truth is nobody wants to be forced into anything—especially change. We resent it when we don't choose our path freely.

I'll bet at some time or another, you've gone to your closet to get dressed and found a pair of pants that no longer fits. This forces you to do one of two things—both of which you are likely to resent. One, you could go out and buy new clothes. Or two, you could go on a diet to lose the extra weight. As a result of being forced into either decision, you likely became resentful. You resent the change that is required to resolve the problem.

My father is an example of someone who was forced to change. He changed the way he ate, exercised, and took care of his body after he had a heart attack. While he was thankful to get a second chance, he did not take up running because it was a pleasurable, proactive way to improve his health. He did it to save his life.

Wouldn't it be better if you chose change not because you had to, but because you care about you? Allowing quality of life—and not crisis—to motivate you makes changing easier, more exciting, and more fun while helping you to avoid unnecessary detours along the way.

TAKE ACTION ON YOUR RESOLUTIONS

How many times have you made a New Year's resolution to lose weight, get in shape, start saving, take a vacation, or spend more time with your loved ones? How long were you able to keep your commitments? Right now, I want you to forget about these previous attempts and start fresh. It doesn't matter whether you've started a dozen diets and stopped, tried to resign from a dead-end job and backed down, or made it only two minutes when you were trying to meditate. This book is going to show you how to put change principles to work for you without all the hesitation or heartbreak any past attempts may have had. I am not going to let you do a last-minute scramble to regain what you could have kept all along.

If you really believe you cannot change the quality of your life today or in the future, then go ahead and close this book. You can just keep doing the same things you always do and getting the same things you always get, or you can allow me to escort you into the best years of your life.

TAKING ADVANTAGE OF THE ODDS

Perhaps you are not ready to believe in the fact that you're likely to see your 100th birthday. You may not even want to live to 100. You may find the thought of it depressing. However, your resistance won't change the fact that your odds of getting there are greater than ever. Very few, if any, of our current centenarians wanted to get there either, but they got there anyway.

It's not enough for me—or the news media—to throw information at you. This will not motivate you to change. You have to want what is rightfully yours. You have to want to be well. It's not enough to simply avoid sickness. You have to want to live the quality life that deep down you know you deserve. Changing your mind about how long you can—and probably will—live opens up a whole world of opportunity. This new paradigm brings better health, fuller coffers, and richer relationships as a result of your acceptance of this wondrous gift. Align yourself with a true view of your potential and it will be hard for anyone or anything to pull you off course.

In a recent *Discover* magazine article, scientists concluded that a child born today has the potential to live 150 years, with some experts asserting that there is no upward limit on your longevity.

Their findings mean living to 100 is not just for a select few, but for you and me as well. It means that evolution and advances in health care and self-care have given you a biological bonus. It is a gift of extra time to accomplish all your goals, nurture your relationships, master your areas of interest, and contribute more to the world. Knowing that you really do have all the time you need to reach your destination could even stop your "urgency addiction" of rushing from one point to the next. It's a gift that can give you the strength and patience to take on even the most challenging opportunities in your life. You still have tons of time to make the necessary changes and enjoy the results of those changes for decades.

How well would you say your biological clock has been keeping time? Are you feeling or looking older than you'd like? Are there aspects of yourself you'd like to change? No matter where you are in your 100-year journey so far, it is not time to slow down or "settle" for any one thing or place in life. But, it is time to get your mind onboard with what you know your body can do and embrace the reality of your longevity with passion.

ADVANCE NOTICE ON AGING

When was the last time you looked through your family photo albums? Take them out and look at your mother and father when they were your age. Look at their parents when they were younger, too. Now think about how they aged. Look at their skin and their posture. How severely did their activity decline as they aged? Did they become crippled by preventable health problems such as arthritis, osteoporosis, or heart disease?

The number of people who are affected by these and many other preventable health conditions is staggering. Twenty million people are affected by osteoarthritis in the United States. Nearly 20 percent of adults older than 65 are obese and another 40 percent are overweight, putting them at substantially increased risk for diabetes, hypertension, heart disease, and other illnesses. Many health conditions that we take for granted in this country are not a normal part of aging elsewhere. They are largely brought on by lifestyle—by our choices. Even universal passages like menopause are simply not the same throughout the world. Japanese women who consume soy as a regular part of their daily diets experience far fewer hot flashes.

The answer, however, isn't to run out and buy soy supplements to treat menopause like a disease. In fact, the usefulness of soy in that form is now a topic for debate. We are talking about your personal lifestyle choices and how they impact you. So, now it's time to take a good look at you. Scan your own reflection in the mirror. How are your skin, bones, and waistline? In what kind of shape are your heart, lungs, liver, and kidneys? Is your spine aligned and is your nervous system functioning to its full potential? If you continue on your current path, will you like the way you age? Can you imagine your photograph in twenty, thirty, or forty years? Embracing The 100-Year Lifestyle will ensure that you blossom over the remaining decades that lie ahead of you.

What did your parents and grandparents know about their own aging potential? When today's centenarians were born, they were only given a life expectancy of 50 years. They were blindsided by their longevity. During their lifetimes, their life expectancies doubled without warning. They had no vision and no strategy for their extended lives. What a surprise it must be for them to find themselves still living. None of them ever thought they could live to 100, but their bodies did it regardless of what they believed. No wonder many of them sit around as grumpy old people. How do you feel when you are a week or a month late on a project? Doesn't this cause you to be angry or frustrated? Can you imagine if you were 30, 40, or 50 years late for your funeral?

This generation that Tom Brokaw called "the Greatest Generation" has lived through World War I and World War II, developed the automobile and airplane, sent humans to the moon, and managed to outlive their predicted life span by five decades! They have watched in disbelief as technology moved center stage— with the advent of the radio, then television, computers, and the Internet. Just as technology has advanced, so has the length of their lives. They have reached record longevity. This in spite of what they thought they knew to be true.

Your grandparents and parents weren't taught that their bodies were designed to live 100 years or more. They weren't taught how to prepare for their longevity. Many of them didn't cultivate physical or financial stability to ensure 100 or more quality years. This "Greatest Generation" is now giving you your greatest gift. They are giving you a preview of what awaits you as a result of your ability to live longer and wiser than any generation before you.

THE ACCIDENTAL CENTENARIANS

The majority of today's centenarians never thought about how they would approach their later years because they never expected to have them. They got there by accident. This "Greatest Generation" is now paying the greatest price for not knowing. In fact, many of them are paying over $10,000 a month to live in nursing homes. They have gone from Greatest Generation to Nursing Home Generation.

These seniors were simply not prepared for such an extended stay here on earth. They believed that if they worked for 35 or 40 years, they could live off of their Social Security benefits, pensions, or retirement funds for their remaining 10 to 20 years maximum, and then they would die. The truth is those resources now need to last twice as long. Our government is grappling with the consequences of this quandary as they are now scrambling to try and save Social Security and Medicare.

What this amounts to is your advance notice. What will you do with this information?

Living the 100-Year Lifestyle   Madame Jeanne Calment lived a 100-Year Lifestyle. She reportedly took up fencing at 85, was still riding her bike at 100, and released a rap CD at 121 years of age. She was still, learning, growing, and staying physically active as she reached and surpassed the 100-year mark.

In search of purpose, passion, and a little extra cash, many seniors are going back to work in the latter part of their lives.

They find the field of opportunity really opens up during their "Second Act" since money is oftentimes no longer their primary motivation.

Older Americans are also heading back to school in droves. Nearly 435,000 Americans 50-plus years of age and older are now part-time college students. Another 120,000 are working toward graduate degrees and 85,000 are full-time college students. Compare this active, happy lifestyle to the 86-year-old mother of a patient of mine. She fell and broke her hip last year. Since then, her health has been declining quickly. Every time the daughter's phone rings, she panics. She knows it will be another issue with her mom. She prays her mother has not broken another hip or lost another ten pounds. She prays she will not grow old the same way her mother has.

> **Centenarian Secret** Aging poorly is not inevitable. You do have a choice. Based on your parents' and grandparents' experiences, you'll see where you're headed unless you choose a different path.

This book is about making choices that will support the quality of your longevity—today and tomorrow. Honor the life you have been given by making the most of the time you have. The fact is that if you are living life to the fullest, maxing out your potential, and enjoying your most important relationships, your life is going to feel pretty short. Even if it lasts beyond 100, it will feel like it is flying by.

Keep your vision in sync with your biology. Calibrate your vision with your extended life span to ensure that the quality matches the quantity of your years. The power of this paradigm shift will give you the ability to write the remaining chapters of your life—with the best ones still to come.

A NEW WAY OF AGING

It's no wonder that so many people have anxiety about aging. *The Merriam-Webster Dictionary* defines it as "a declining phase of life." However, today's pre- and post-centenarians are reinventing our notion of aging. Like former U.S. President George H. W. Bush who celebrated his 70th birthday by going skydiving, many seniors are pushing the limits of their genetic potential and loving every minute of it, realizing that they have plenty of time left to live their life!

Today's centenarians are teaching us that growing older is not a one-way ticket to deterioration and inactivity. They are showing us a new way of aging that is full of excitement and opportunity if you combine the right attitude with the right actions.

Living the 100-Year Lifestyle: Gene Pollack   Gene Pollock is 83 years old and has enjoyed over 20 careers over his lifetime—as a paint salesman, and then a WWII fighter pilot, a forest ranger, motion picture actor, screenwriter, college professor, Golden Glove boxer, and an artist. The secret to his longevity is his mental outlook and the opportunities he attracts. He embraces change. He sees every new experience as enriching his life and he has learned to have no regrets when life says it's time to move on. He has allowed change to fuel and charge his life with positive experiences. This is the essence of the 100-Year Lifestyle.

How do you feel about your experience so far? Would a change of personal habits, residence, relationships, career, health, or finances improve your level of happiness and prosperity? Will the choices you have made so far enable you to look back with no regrets when you are 80, 90, or 100?

I know you know the things you need to change. "Yes," you say, "I know it is easier to be fit than fat. I know it is easier to be solvent than bankrupt. I know it is better to be in love than alone." But, what are you doing with what you know? Don't you think it's time to stop just thinking about it and to start acting on change? You do have time to turn things around and take things to the next level. Let's get started.

CHAPTER 2
THE THREE LIFE-CHANGING PRINCIPLES OF THE 100-YEAR LIFESTYLE

Are you still with me? Great. You are on your way to living your best life, every day of your life, for 100 years and beyond. We'll begin by embracing the changes you know you need to make. In the chapters ahead, you'll discover how to access the energy to fuel your longevity while ending all the old habits, patterns, and behaviors that are keeping you from living your best life every day. You will then become healthier than you've ever been before and put a team in place to sustain that health for a lifetime. Next, you'll create an ideal environment and support system for your extended life and set yourself up to enjoy the journey more than ever. You'll learn how to achieve balance, finance your 100-Year Lifestyle, and enjoy your best life every step of the way.

At the core of customizing your 100-Year Lifestyle are three life-changing principles that you will use throughout this journey:

Change Principle #1:
Change is easy. Thinking about change is hard.

Change Principle #2:
Change happens one choice at a time. Think progress, not perfection.

Change Principle #3:
Approach change with your ideal 100-Year Lifestyle in mind.

These principles will make change exciting and achievable. They will empower you to age constructively instead of destructively. They will help you make your life so much more than before because the odds are you are going to have nearly a century or more to mold your life into everything you've always wanted it to be.

CHANGE PRINCIPLE #1
CHANGE IS EASY—THINKING ABOUT CHANGE IS HARD

You've probably already experienced this: Resisting change is much harder than embracing it.

If you've ever played with magnets, you can understand the power behind Change Principle #1. When you hold two magnets near each other with the like poles pointed toward each other, they repel one another no matter how hard you try to make the two ends meet. However, once you flip their orientation so the opposite charges are facing each other, they effortlessly attract and stick together. Then, instead of requiring energy to hold them together, it takes enormous energy to pull the magnets apart.

The magnet experiment is a metaphor for how we experience change once we commit to it. I see this play out in my patients and clients who continue with bad habits that force them to expend excess energy just to keep their lives together—knowing that it would be less effort if they just went ahead and chose a healthier path. I love watching the pieces of their lives fall effortlessly into place once they commit to change. It is a physical demonstration of Change Principle #1 and how change is easy. It's the thinking about it that is hard.

Centenarian Secret Resisting the things you know you need to change polarizes your life. This keeps you stuck. However, when you embrace change, the pieces of your life will fall naturally into place and stay there, just like the magnets.

What do you want to change? Do you want to be thinner, smarter, better paid, more loved, or healthier? What will you do to attract these things with ease? It's time to flip your mental magnet. Let your quest for quality and not crisis motivate you if you are ready to upgrade to your ideal 100 Year-Lifestyle.

While you are in the process of thinking about what you want to change, your life may look and feel difficult. In fact, vacillating between crisis and quality-of-life motivation mode can keep you on an emotional roller coaster—with respect to your health, your marriage, your kids, and your finances. But, once you've made the commitment to change—and I mean *really* made it—then you will find that many of the things you have been struggling with will fall easily into place. Activities and choices that aren't in alignment with creating your best life will lose their appeal. Like flipping the magnet, you will begin to attract the people and resources you need to reach your greatest dreams and goals once you shift your belief about what you think you can accomplish. Whether it is health for 100 years or undying passion for your family or a hobby, you get to decide what happens in the second half of your journey—one choice at a time.

This resistance to change is something I observed time and again over the past 20 years, as I worked with thousands of patients to help them heal and maximize the quality of their lives. One of my patients was a successful stockbroker named Jim. About twice a year, Jim would come in for "crisis care" when he was experiencing severe episodes of back pain. Each time, I would encourage him to change his life by correcting the under-lying problem rather than slapping a "Band-Aid" on his symp-toms. Jim would always respond by telling me that he knew I was right, but that he "just didn't have the time to commit to it." When I asked Jim if he had time for his current crisis, he would laugh and say, "Of course not," but he wasn't interested in chang-ing his routine.

Over the years, the episodes would get more painful, more expensive, and more inconvenient for Jim. Each time he came in, we would talk about how much better it would be if he allowed quality of life to motivate his health choices instead of crisis. Finally, after years of deteriorating health and one inconvenient crisis after another, Jim committed to change. He made taking care of his back and spending more time with his family a priority. Two years later, he was happier and healthier than I had ever seen him. "I feel young and energetic again," he said. His business was better than ever, his marriage was better than ever, and he was playing more golf (and better golf) than ever. He was truly enjoying the best of his life.

Jim's quality of life was lousy when he was just thinking about changing it, but once he finally committed to making the changes he knew he needed to make and made those changes his lifestyle, he began to magnetically attract great things into his life naturally.

CHANGE PRINCIPLE #2
CHANGE HAPPENS ONE CHOICE AT TIME—THINK PROGRESS, NOT PERFECTION

As you learn how to make the changes that will support your best life today and in the future, remember that you may not see results right away.

One of the principles of change is that it occurs over time. We "titrate" into it slowly. I've borrowed the term *titration* from the chemistry experiment most of us conducted in school. You know the one. It was the lesson where your teacher gave you a glass beaker filled with a clear liquid and a dropper with another chemical solution. You were asked to take the chemical and drop it into the beaker one drop at a time and record how many drops it took to change the liquid's color. Do you remember how nothing happened at first? You would drop, drop, drop and it would still be clear, but then suddenly, one last drop, and the liquid's color would instantly change!

In the process of chemical titration, you are determining the exact number of drops necessary to produce the desired effect or change in the solution. The question many students found themselves asking was which drop was the most important? Some believed it was the first drop because it began the transformation. Others thought it was the last one because that's the one where they actually saw the liquid change color. The truth is that they are all of equal importance, because without any one of them, the solution would not have changed.

This is how the results from the changes you make often appear. You have to lose one pound at a time before you finally shed 50. You have to walk a minute before you can make it a mile. Change arrives one input at a time, one choice at a time. It is an accumulation of actions that will color your life with joy or suffering—depending upon the quality of your choices.

What kind of commitment and actions do you think it will take before you start seeing the rewards of your efforts?

You can never be sure how many "drops" or acts of changed behavior it will take to get you to your desired destination. This is why you must approach change with a healthy attitude—acknowledging progress without sabotaging your own success by demanding perfection. What you can be sure of, though, is this: The color and quality of your life will fade if you always choose to let crisis be your motivating force.

Now that you know it's possible to live a century or longer, how will you spend the rest of your years? What kind of drops will you add to your life each day? Will you wear out your body in the first 40, 50, or 60 years, or be like Jack LaLanne and entertain the idea of swimming across a large body of water when you have a milestone birthday? The truth is, you don't get to choose how and when you are going to die, but you can choose how you're going to live. By changing your life today and making those changes your lifestyle, you will impact the level of health and prosperity (or suffering) you experience as you age.

Each choice you make will build momentum for the future while giving you confidence and enthusiasm in the present. Remember, when you choose, you are either choosing to stay on the path of your ideal 100-Year Lifestyle, or you are choosing something else. If you are going to make progress at something over the next 20, 30, or 40 years, why not make progress toward the things that you value the most. Every choice that would improve your life when you are 100 would also improve your life today.

Many of us make toxic choices that limit our life. In fact, they often come disguised as rewards. For instance, have you ever reached for a cigarette as a reward at the end of a hard day or downed another dessert as an emotional pick-me-up? Were the five minutes of enjoyment worth the three days of guilt and two weeks of trying to get back on track? Your true reward comes from the self-esteem and love you give yourself when you honor yourself with each choice.

Centenarian Secret   Your ideal 100-Year Lifestyle choices are the ones that will not only positively impact your life today, but when you are 60, 70, 80, 90, or 100.

Make the rest of your life the best of your life. Learn how to commit to and then recommit to what you need to change. If you want to be nicotine-free, you have to make that commitment and then recommit to it every minute of every day. If you want to save money, then you have to make that commitment and recommit to walking away from empty purchases each day. If you want to be healthy and fit, then prove it to yourself every day with each choice.

If you find yourself getting off track from your goals, it's okay. Think progress, not perfection. You can gently nudge yourself back on track with your next choice knowing you are in the process of building the lifestyle you can enjoy for 100 years.

CHANGE PRINCIPLE #3
APPROACH CHANGE WITH YOUR IDEAL 100-YEAR LIFESTYLE IN MIND

Welcome to Change Principle #3. It's time to go for the gold, whatever that means to you, as you start approaching your life with a fresh, new expectation in mind and develop an exciting vision for the rest of your life. It is a shift that will allow you to keep your brains, your looks, your possessions, and your mojo as you age. It is a shift that will allow you to live your ideal 100-Year Lifestyle without compromise. It is time to draw a line in the sand and declare that the balance of your life will be the most fun, exciting, and fulfilling times you have ever experienced.

A few years ago, I had a patient who needed to lose weight. Bill was a former athlete but he had committed so much time to his marriage, raising his kids, and working that his health had declined slowly over time. He worked hard at getting rid of his extra weight, but it never seemed to stay off. As he dieted, he constantly focused on what he could not have. He felt very restricted and disliked the taste of many low-fat substitutes. The process was slow and unsatisfying. I knew he needed and wanted to change.

One day, I sat Bill down and helped him see how losing weight wasn't about *losing* anything at all. I explained that his choice to trim down meant he was really *gaining* muscle, energy, and self-esteem. He was building a stronger heart and overall health. His goals seemed more attainable when he changed his focus. He approached his new nutrition and lifestyle habits not from a belief that he was losing something, but from a belief that he was gaining a life that he could really be excited about. So he made the changes he knew he needed to make, and 30 days later when he came in for his appointment wearing exercise clothes and looking "fast and fit," as he said, he was feeling younger than he had felt in 25 years.

Just as change that focuses on "loss" can be hard to sustain, so is change that results in lateral movement. One of my colleagues was struggling in her practice and decided to close up shop and reopen in a different town. She changed her location, but she never expanded her skill set or changed how she practiced health care. Her new practice ended up just like the old one—with the same old problems as the ones she tried to leave behind.

She was not able to create a better practice because her focus was not in the right place. She made a sideways move that caused a superficial shift and the same stressful practice. Instead, she might have looked at how the health care industry was changing, how to improve the quality of her care, or how the needs of her patients were evolving. You see this happen with people again and again—not just professionally, but even in terms of their relationships. People take knee-jerk actions without slowing down and taking time to consider the true nature of a problem. In the case of my colleague, she approached change not with her ideal 100-Year Lifestyle, but with the idea of escaping the mistakes she had made in her old location. It was an approach that kept her stuck in her old destructive patterns.

Centenarian Secret   Approaching change with your ideal 100-Year Lifestyle in mind is the key to creating results. This is how you will optimize the quality and quantity of your life. It is the only focus that will keep you consistently motivated during your "titration" process—as you get from where you are to where you want to be.

With this knowledge, you now have the opportunity to make the changes that will lead you toward an incredible 100-Year Lifestyle. You may be wondering where to start. What are the means for getting to this end? How much money will you want? How will you nurture your marriage and other relationships over this extended period of time?

The questions I've developed for you at the end of this chapter will help you begin to personalize and prioritize your plan. First, you need to get in touch with what you really want and deserve. This can be difficult, particularly when it is out of step with the values of your family or peer group. However, if that's the case, you've been more of a follower than a leader and it's time to take back the reins. Now is your time to step up and take charge. You'll soon see that you will not only start creating positive change in your own life, but also in the lives of people around you. You'll be a healthy influence. Expect some relationships to deepen and some to fall away. You will open the door to magnetically attracting support for your 100-Year Lifestyle. As you begin to customize your vision, don't settle. Dare yourself. Stretch yourself. Go for the goal that burns brightest in your gut.

Expect progress—not perfection—as you embark on this new path that I will guide you on throughout this book. Although you don't have complete control over how long you'll live, you've got control over the quality of those years. Assume you are here for a reason. Spend your days discovering that reason. Relax into the ebb and flow of life. Trust yourself and begin to connect with your core like never before. Find the meaning and opportunity in everything. When you do that, the length of your life doesn't matter anyway. The ultimate question will be whether you fulfilled your purpose and lived your life to the fullest and without regret.

In the chapters ahead, you'll customize your 100-Year Lifestyle. You'll learn how to live longer, become wiser, optimize your environment, eliminate stress, and establish routines, relationships, and learning patterns that will support you in that lifestyle. You will capitalize on time (since you are going to have so much more of it than you thought), extend your income, and build a compass for lasting purpose.

Now let's get specific and personal.

▶ LIVE LONG AND STRONG EXERCISE
In each of the following areas, what are the changes you want to make with your ideal 100-Year Lifestyle in mind:

- » Your health?
- » Your environment?
- » Your schedule?
- » Your finances?
- » Your relationships?
- » Your career?
- » How you spend your free time?
- » How you use your talents?
- » How you manage stress?
- » The way you treat people? Or how you allow them to treat you?
- » The way you think about your past?
- » The way you approach your future?

Make these changes your lifestyle.

Choose up to three areas that are the most important to you. Commit to change. Then, be prepared to recommit to it every time your choice is challenged.

Remember, staying the same will be harder than just making the change. Your hesitation is what keeps you on the emotional roller coaster. All that emotional energy is spent and you produce nothing. You find yourself right back in your old patterns and issues.

Whether it's exercising more, eating healthier, or managing your time and money better—make choices with your 100-Year Lifestyle in mind. You will improve your life tomorrow and improve your life today while you balance your desire for immediate gratification with your long-term desires. Always keep in mind the future that you want to experience—this will ensure that the quality of your years keeps pace with the quantity of time you have left.

It's time to declare your vision for the next phase of your life. What will your last decade be like? Whether you live to 70, 80, 90, or 100-plus, the choices you make today will define the depth and breadth of what you experience tomorrow.

Don't worry about whether you'll have the strength and discipline to follow through on your 100-Year Lifestyle. One day at a time, one choice at a time, we'll do it together and, God willing, enjoy a sensational century.

Turn the page now and find the energy to change with the excitement of knowing you are just getting started. The fun has just begun.

THE 100-YEAR LIFESTYLE
ACTION PLAN FOR LASTING CHANGE

1. *Take Advantage of the Advanced Notice.*
   Listen to the advanced notice your parents and grandparents are giving you about how long you can and probably will live. Make life choices for the long haul. Start planning your 100-Year Lifestyle today, so you can experience a life of

lasting health, wealth, prosperity, partnership, and purpose as you age.

2. *Put the Three Life-Changing Principles to Work for You.*
   These principles represent the simple truth about change that can keep you consistently committed to the changes you know you want and need to make.

3. *Change Is Easy—Thinking about Change Is Hard.*
   Change happens one choice at a time. Think progress, not perfection. Approach change with your ideal 100-Year Lifestyle in mind.

4. *Choose Quality-of-Life Motivation—Not Crisis Motivation.*
   Allowing crisis to motivate you to change keeps you in your old patterns and issues. Choose quality of life motivation over the crisis approach to change. That way, you'll avoid many painful, unnecessary detours along the way.

5. *Choose up to Three Areas to Change.*
   What are the priority areas of your life you want to change? Whether it's your health, your finances, your work, or relationships, choose up to three and start titrating change into them today. Lasting change is easy when you allow yourself to build momentum.

6. *Approach Change with Your Ideal 100-Year Lifestyle in Mind.*
   Watch your focus. Question whether the choices you make today could be temporary gains or toxic solutions. Your best life choices are ones that will positively impact your life both today and when you are 60, 70, 80, 90, or 100. This focus will give you a foundation of clear and lasting commitment to becoming the best you.

7. *The Rest of Your Life Can Be the Best of Your Life.*
   Dare yourself! Make it a sensational century. Live and leave your best life legacy as you learn how to live longer, healthier, and wiser than any other generation in history.

Life Expectancy at Birth by Race and Sex, 1930–2002

YEAR	ALL RACES BOTH SEXES	MALE	FEMALE	WHITE BOTH SEXES	MALE	FEMALE	BLACK BOTH SEXES	MALE	FEMALE
2002	77.3	74.5	79.9	77.7	75.1	80.3	72.3	68.8	75.6
2001	77.2	74.4	79.8	77.7	75.0	80.2	72.2	68.6	75.5
2000	77.0	74.3	79.7	77.6	74.9	80.1	71.9	68.3	75.2
1999	76.7	73.9	79.4	77.3	74.6	79.9	71.4	67.8	74.7
1998	76.7	73.8	79.5	77.3	74.5	80.0	71.3	67.6	74.8
1997	76.5	73.6	79.4	77.2	74.3	79.9	71.1	67.2	74.7
1996	76.1	73.1	79.1	76.8	73.9	79.7	70.2	66.1	74.2
1995	75.8	72.5	78.9	76.5	73.4	79.6	69.6	65.2	73.9
1994	75.7	72.4	79.0	76.5	73.3	79.6	69.5	64.9	73.9
1993	75.5	72.2	78.8	76.3	73.1	79.5	69.2	64.6	73.7
1992	75.8	72.3	79.1	76.5	73.2	79.8	69.6	65.0	73.9
1991	75.5	72.0	78.9	76.3	72.9	79.6	69.3	64.6	73.8
1990	75.4	71.8	78.8	76.1	72.7	79.4	69.1	64.5	73.6
1989	75.1	71.7	78.5	75.9	72.5	79.2	68.8	64.3	73.3
1988	74.9	71.4	78.3	75.6	72.2	78.9	68.9	64.4	73.2
1987	74.9	71.4	78.3	75.6	72.1	78.9	69.1	64.7	73.4
1986	74.7	71.2	78.2	75.4	71.9	78.8	69.1	64.8	73.4
1985	74.7	71.1	78.2	75.3	71.8	78.7	69.3	65.0	73.4
1984	74.7	71.1	78.2	75.3	71.8	78.7	69.5	65.3	73.6
1983	74.6	71.0	78.1	75.2	71.6	78.7	69.4	65.2	73.5
1982	74.5	70.8	78.1	75.1	71.5	78.7	69.4	65.1	73.6
1981	74.1	70.4	77.8	74.8	71.1	78.4	68.9	64.5	73.2

Life Expectancy at Birth by Race and Sex, 1930–2002

	ALL RACES			WHITE			BLACK		
YEAR	BOTH SEXES	MALE	FEMALE	BOTH SEXES	MALE	FEMALE	BOTH SEXES	MALE	FEMALE
1980	73.7	70.0	77.4	74.4	70.7	78.1	68.1	63.8	72.5
1979	73.9	70.0	77.8	74.6	70.8	78.4	68.5	64.0	72.9
1978	73.5	69.6	77.3	74.1	70.4	78.0	68.1	63.7	72.4
1977	73.3	69.5	77.2	74.0	70.2	77.9	67.7	63.4	72.0
1976	72.9	69.1	76.8	73.6	69.9	77.5	67.2	62.9	71.6
1975	72.6	68.8	76.6	73.4	69.5	77.3	66.8	62.4	71.3
1974	72.0	68.2	75.9	72.8	69.0	76.7	66.0	61.7	70.3
1973	71.4	67.6	75.3	72.2	68.5	76.1	65.0	60.9	69.3
1972	71.2	67.4	75.1	72.0	68.3	75.9	64.7	60.4	69.1
1971	71.1	67.4	75.0	72.0	68.3	75.8	64.6	60.5	68.9
1970	70.8	67.1	74.7	71.7	68.0	75.6	64.1	60.0	68.3
1960	69.7	66.6	73.1	70.6	67.4	74.1	—	—	—
1950	68.2	65.6	71.1	69.1	66.5	72.2	—	—	—
1940	62.9	60.8	65.2	64.2	62.1	66.6	—	—	—
1935	61.7	59.9	63.9	62.9	61.0	65.0	53.1	51.1	55.2
1930	59.7	58.1	61.6	61.4	59.7	63.5	48.1	47.3	49.2

Table Information

(—) Data not available

Figures are revised

Deaths based on a 50 percent sample

Source: National Center for Health Statistics, National Vital Statistics
Reports, vol. 52, no. 3, 18 September, 2003. Web: www.cdc.gov/nchs

PART 2

Enjoying Youthful Energy at Every Age

Wherever you focus your energy, that's where it goes.

CHAPTER 3
FINDING THE ENERGY TO CHANGE YOUR LIFE

If you're ready to start living a 100-Year Lifestyle but aren't sure you've got the energy for it, I've got some exciting news for you. It's not your age that's exhausting you. It's how you choose to utilize your energy. Your focus either wears you out or wakes you up. Wherever you focus your energy, it goes.

If your life is anything like mine, you probably operate at a fast pace. In fact, thinking about changing your schedule or commitments may seem even more exhausting than the clip you maintain to keep up. That's why so many of us unintentionally use crisis to create the extra energy we need to justify changing our lives. We don't intend to stay in the status quo or rob ourselves of a 100-Year Lifestyle. Yet, somehow we end up on autopilot.

Why we do it is unique to each of us. Some of us lack drive. Some of us love the familiar. Maybe we are comfortable. The reasons really aren't that important. The truth is that change is a high-energy investment that appreciates over time and the good news is that your energy to change already exists. The question is, Where have you been spending it?

I was recently coaching a doctor who was unhappy with his practice. He wanted to make a change. Managed care had hurt his profitability. His practice felt more like a burden than a joy. Though he was an excellent healer, he was losing the passion he once had for his work. When I began suggesting what he could do to make his vocation fun and exciting again, I was shocked by his reaction. He began to argue with me, insisting that it wasn't possible. He focused on why he couldn't make the changes he knew he needed to make.

His face got red. His posture became defensive. There was an edge in his voice. The amount of energy he expended to defend why he couldn't change was incredible. He ran down a list of at least ten different reasons why things had to stay the same. Five minutes into the conversation, I felt more like I was in a courtroom with a defense attorney rather than a coaching session. He had built a tremendous case against himself, defending why he couldn't change. I was listening to some of the negative chatter that played inside his head, day after day. The chatter was, in large part, unconscious.

A few days later, I was talking with a patient who was a very successful entrepreneur. Her all-work, no-play routine was taking a toll on her health and her family. She was exhausted. Her back hurt, and her level of stress was off the charts. When I suggested she take some time for herself, she began to argue with me, listing the reasons why she couldn't. Her clients wouldn't like it, she told me. Her cell phone, in fact, interrupted our conversation a few times and we had to constantly start over again. It was tiring just watching her. This woman is a great salesperson and she could sell anything to anybody. Her challenge was that she had sold herself on the fact that she couldn't change. And she was wasting a lot of energy in the process. No wonder she was stuck and exhausted.

I asked these two people, who were having trouble finding the energy to change, the same question that I am about to ask you: Whose side are you on, anyway?

They soon discovered, as you will too, that one of the places where the energy to change springs from is the decision to stop defending why you can't change. What would happen if you started to build a case for why you could live your ideal 100-Year Lifestyle, instead of investing your energy in arguing why you can't? After all, like it or not, you may have 30, 40, 50, or even 60 years before you reach 100. Your newfound energy would come from the same place it comes from now, only you will use it differently. You would use it to support, encourage, and take action to make the rest of your life the best. Your energy level would skyrocket.

HOW TO MASTER CHANGE

Remember Change Principle #1: *Change is easy. Thinking about change is hard.* In the long run, staying the same often requires more energy than changing. When you don't make the changes you know you need to make, your energy is wasted on survival, boredom, anger, and frustration—that creates stress, worry, anxiety, and other energy-draining emotions. When you recognize it, you can consciously begin to change the way you expend your energy to restore your enthusiasm, health, success, and vigor.

What would you do if you were to suffer from a disability? Would you stay in the safety of your wheelchair or tackle the world and embrace your challenges? Would you play the victim and defend your limitations with all your energy or would you build the case for why you can overcome them, be healthy, and live your unique 100-Year Lifestyle?

One of the reasons thinking about change (Change Principle #1) is so hard is because it eats up your energy and produces fear. Many of us fear change because we are afraid of how other people will react. Often, it seems easier to stay where we are. But when you choose change and commit to it, you'll find in time that your own certainty and confidence surpasses those fears and doubts and gets you moving forward. You begin to magnetically attract support as the people around you realize that you are serious and committed to your new life.

As you saw with Kyle, this can happen slowly over time or it can happen the instant you truly decide without looking back.

Quite often, the reasons why you think you can't change are the reasons why you can, should, and must. If you think you can't find the time to exercise because you've got to take the kids to school, cook dinner, and pay the bills, then that's the reason why you should. If you don't, you are shorting both yourself and your family by giving them a partial you—someone who is exhausted, edgy, and resentful all the time.

▶ LIVING THE 100-YEAR LIFESTYLE:

Kyle Maynard

One of my patients, 19-year-old Kyle Maynard, knows what I'm talking about.

You may have seen Kyle on *ESPN*, *Larry King Live*, in *USA Today*, or in one of the many other magazines that have featured his story. Kyle was born without full limbs. They were missing just below the elbow and knee. Standing only two and a half feet tall and weighing 123 pounds, this courageous young athlete chose to join his school wrestling team at the age of 11.

Most people thought what he was attempting to do was impossible. But his parents supported his determination to learn the sport. Kyle, who walks and runs on all fours, spent hours practicing each day. But his first 35 matches were losses.

As a sophomore and junior, Kyle finally titrated into winning. By his senior year, his record of 35-16 placed him in the top 12 in Georgia and the top 12 in the nationals. A broken nose is all that kept him from being named All American in 2004. Today, Kyle is an invaluable member of the University of Georgia wrestling team, a best-selling author of the book *No Excuses*, and a mighty motivational speaker.

How has he overpowered his wrestling opponents? He triumphs because, believe it or not, his challengers see him as having the advantage. His opponents believe Kyle's small stature makes him swifter and stronger than they are. What an irony that someone with congenitally amputated arms and legs could have the upper hand!

Many of us use "what's missing" in our lives as the reason for why we can't change or why we can't reach our goals. "Instead of telling people what I am going to try to do, I just go out and do it," says Kyle. "Once they see it, then they believe it can be done." Kyle makes no excuses for why he "can't" achieve. He doesn't wait for permission to be told what he can or can't do.

Change Happens One Choice at a Time

Right now, I would like you to think of one thing you would like to change. For example, maybe the family budget feels a little tight and you'd like a little extra money. Maybe you just retired from a position you held for 25 years and you are looking for something new to which you can commit. Maybe you are suffering from a health problem and need to heal. No matter what type of change you may be contemplating, ask yourself these questions:

Who are the people in your life who can support you in reaching your goals?

What experiences and skills do you already have to get where you want to go?

From here, start to design a plan. But be prepared to take things step by step. Think progress, not perfection (Change Principle #2).

Centenarian Secret   Great things happen when you have the wherewithal to stick to your commitment to change. You find yourself respected by people you respect. You create a life story that inspires other people. You show other people what is possible. Have the grit to see it through. Go for your ideal 100-Year Lifestyle. If not now, when? How many more decades will you compromise yourself about what you know innately is right for you?

Now, obviously starting a revenue-generating business is one of the most complicated changes you can make—especially one that makes you a multimillionaire. But it's very possible when you make one choice at a time with your ideal 100-Year Lifestyle in mind.

As you read through the rest of this book, you'll find additional tools and strategies to help you create successful change. You can count on me to show you how to stock your mind and body with the energy and power to make these changes you know you need to make. Understand, though, that to create change, *you* will need to change. You must start doing things differently. You can't always go with the flow—sometimes you have to let go.

Joyce Bone

Joyce Bone, the mother of a newborn, was in her late twenties, living in Atlanta. She had worked for a while but left the corporate world to start her family. As a result, she and her husband had gone from two incomes to one. One day, she was taking her baby for a walk in a stroller while listening to an inspirational cassette. The question came up, "If your life was exactly how you would like it to be, what would it look like?"

Joyce says, "I remember thinking at the time that I had a great life—a beautiful child, a large and supportive family, and a handsome husband. The one thing we could have used was a little more money. Our family budget was a little tight."

While she was nervous about making the call, she soon contacted her old boss. Ten days later, they got together and had lunch. She explained her desires and together they explored possible ways of teaming up and working together again. At this stage, her boss was more of an "ideas" person and an investor. Joyce was at a place in her life where she was more hands-on. They began to conceive of a business idea that day at lunch, which they hashed out on a napkin at the restaurant. They decided to team up in the male-dominated liquid-waste industry. Joyce would run a business. Her boss would arrange financing for the acquisition of a company.

"Eighteen months later, I went from a stay-at-home mom to CEO of a business employing 350 employees and generating $50 million in revenue," she says. Her very first day on the job, she was asked by one of her male employees to make some copies. Imagine his embarrassment when he soon learned that she was not his new assistant, but his new CEO.

"We went public within two years and my financial goals were met. I retired in my early thirties as a millionaire. It felt like winning the lottery. It was a time of tremendous change. I am still changing because of it."

ENERGY DRAINERS VERSUS ENERGY ENHANCERS

Your energy is one of your most valuable resources, so be selective about how and where you focus it. Don't waste a drop. High-energy potential is your natural state. But you only have so much in a given day. Stress and other distractions can easily deplete this gift if you allow them to drain you. Every decision you make regarding your health, relationships, business, exercise, diet, emotional reactions, and achievements either positively or negatively impacts your energy.

Centenarian Secret   According to the laws of physics, energy can neither be created nor destroyed. This rule, known as the Law of Conservation, says that there is a constant and finite amount of energy in the world. This energy can be converted, however, to produce the outcomes you desire.

This is what happens when we bounce a ball. When you hold a ball above the ground, it has potential energy to fall. When you release the ball, and it begins to move, the energy becomes kinetic. Kinetic energy changes the ball's momentum. Electrical energy from a battery can be converted into mechanical energy to move your car. A small amount of nuclear energy can light the night sky across an entire city.

Have you ever noticed how when you're on fire about a project, your energy soars in much the same way? When you connect with your deepest human potential, you fuel your efforts with a type of kinetic energy that gives you the momentum to transform.

You can reach your goals with your current energy supply if you are willing to redistribute the way you choose to use it. Everyday choices will either support or undermine your human potential. Choose wisely. Do this by distancing yourself from people or situations that deplete you. For me, drinking too much caffeine and not exercising drains my energy. Going for walks and spending time with my spouse and children enhances it.

Now is the time to become your own personal energy manager. You will immediately feel younger and healthier than you have in a long time—regardless of your age. After all, high energy is your natural state. How you choose to use your energy is up to you.

When you master your own energy, you can maintain that high state of energy. You can avoid radical highs and lows. Like programming your home to a comfortable temperature so that the air conditioner turns on when it gets too hot or the heat turns on when it's too cold, you can program your own energy level for consistently high output.

TAKE AN ENERGY INVENTORY

Energy drainers and energy enhancers are very personal. What may be an energy drainer for one person may be an energy enhancer for another. I remember participating in a board meeting where the topic was the bylaws of the organization. The lawyers in the group were passionately debating every word. In the thick of it, my colleague grinned at me and said, "I love this." What was energizing for him was exhausting and draining for me. I kept looking at my watch, counting the seconds as I felt the energy being zapped from my body, while he kept leaping back into the conversation and picking up steam.

Shopping is another activity that energizes some and depletes others. Some people just love "the hunt" and they are captivated by everything that is shiny and new. Others are more focused on the crowds, rude salespeople, and the challenge of tracking down what they really need. However, there are many activities that universally charge us up or deplete us. Most people are energized by quality time with family and friends, or reading a good book. On the other hand, some universal energy drainers include overworking, overeating, and drinking too much alcohol.

Once you take your personal energy inventory, you can consciously begin to make choices that support your high-energy 100-Year Lifestyle. Eliminate the things that drain you. Focus on the things that energize you. When you do this, you will find that you innately have the resources you need to change your life. In fact, not making the change is an energy drainer. The commitment to change ignites a spark for instant energy. Recommitting to that change provides you with a continual feed. For example, if you detest shopping in stores, hire someone to shop for you, or consider shopping online. These days, you can buy most everything you need this way. And doing so frees up time to pursue a potential business idea, play with your children or grandchildren, or plan a special occasion with your spouse.

In the box to the right is a sample list of activities that will measure how well you are using your potential energy. It will help you identify the quality of the choices you are making as they relate to your energy, and whether they are helping or hurting you. Each action is either a credit or debit toward your energy bank. Use your answers to help you shift your energy to live your ideal 100-Year Lifestyle.

Every energy drain has an energy enhancer that can take its place. You just have to train yourself to make that choice. Very often, we find the energy to change by avoiding the activities, habits, and patterns that drain us. Not doing can be just as important as doing.

How you think can also be an energy drainer or an energy enhancer. If worry is a big energy drain for you, try turning your worry into faith. Recently, after going through this exercise with one of my clients, she told me that over the last 30 years of her adult life, she worried all the time. "Nothing that I ever worried about ever happened, but it took so much of my energy. I have so much energy now, sometimes I feel like I don't even need to sleep." Turning worry into faith and strengthening your ability to accept things you cannot change will free up a tremendous amount of your energy. One great saying to help you let go is the Serenity Prayer: "God give me the serenity to accept the things I cannot change, the courage to change the things I can, and the wisdom to know the difference." This is a great mantra if one of your energy leaks is trying to control other people.

After all, worry never made a deposit into a bank account, healed a disease, or changed the weather. Converting worry into an energy-enhancing attitude can free you to direct your energy

▶ LIVE LONG AND STRONG EXERCISE

Check off the statements below that apply to you.

MY ENERGY DRAINERS:
- ❏ Sugar
- ❏ Caffeine
- ❏ Not exercising
- ❏ Arguing with my spouse
- ❏ Stress
- ❏ Drama
- ❏ Interruptions
- ❏ Being overweight
- ❏ Overscheduling my day
- ❏ Saying yes when I mean no
- ❏ Overworking
- ❏ Not taking play time
- ❏ Taking abuse
- ❏ Worry
- ❏ Slouching
- ❏ Overanalyzing
- ❏ Trying to change other people
- ❏ Being a people pleaser
- ❏ Stressing out
- ❏ Mindless television
- ❏ Not having a purpose
- ❏ Not completing things that I start

MY ENERGY ENHANCERS:
- ❏ Speaking my truth
- ❏ Quality time with kids
- ❏ Being honest
- ❏ Following through
- ❏ Reading good books
- ❏ Keeping promises to myself
- ❏ Being grateful
- ❏ Prayer
- ❏ Eating healthy
- ❏ Taking my supplements
- ❏ Date night with spouse
- ❏ Quality time with friends
- ❏ Focusing on the positive
- ❏ Having faith
- ❏ Expressing gratitude
- ❏ Standing up for myself
- ❏ Staying on task
- ❏ Letting go of the things that are out of my control
- ❏ Taking action on my goals
- ❏ Making time to exercise
- ❏ Getting chiropractic care
- ❏ Good posture
- ❏ Massages
- ❏ Saving money
- ❏ Being involved in things I believe in
- ❏ Celebrating special occasions

On what types of activities do you spend most of your time? Do you tend to do things that fuel you? Or do you find that most of your time is spent on activities that deplete you? Your personal energy inventory is a reality check on where your energy is being distributed. I don't want you to perceive it as a list of problems, or a way to defend why things are the way they are. Instead, it is a way to raise your awareness about where all your energy is going and how to get it flowing back into your life.

toward powering change. As you feel your energy grow, it will enhance your creative spirit and set you on the path that will bring you all of the answers and resources to drive your fun, exciting, adventurous 100-Year Lifestyle. You will no longer dread the changes you know you need to make and you will take action. You might consider reading a book on a subject you are passionate about, booking a trip that you have always wanted to take, getting back in to see your nutritionist, chiropractor, or personal trainer to get on a new self-care routine, or decide to let go of your need to control. It's your list. Trust yourself to know what is best for you.

▶ **YOUR PERSONAL ENERGY INVENTORY**

On the left side of this box, list your most draining personal energy drainers. On the right side of this box, list your most enhancing energy enhancers. Add to this list every day as you go through your day and experience things that wear you down or inspire your energy. Once your list is complete, live on the right side of this box and sustain youthful energy regardless of your age.

ENERGY DRAINERS   ENERGY ENHANCERS

EMPLOY ENERGY ENHANCERS

Theoretically, we watch television to entertain ourselves. But quite often, the television set becomes a comfortable diversion—from an exhausting workday, a rude salesclerk, or a family problem. The latter makes television an energy drain. After dinner, when many people settle in with two scoops of ice cream and the remote, you might try going for a power walk, PowerCentering, Pilates, or gardening. You will feel incredible energy doing activities like this and you will sleep better. As a result, you will feel more energized the next day.

Taking a sauna, doing yoga, and drinking a lot of water are also excellent ways to set up a restorative sleep. Other energy-enhancing ideas include walking with neighbors and inviting friends over. You know what energizes and fills you with positive energy better than anyone else. Seek out and fill your life with these choices, and make this your lifestyle. Don't be afraid to vary them—mixing them up is a great way to optimize their benefits and keep things fresh.

Replenish your energy bank one choice at a time (Change Principle #2) by saying "no" to the attitudes and actions that drain your energy and "yes" to the energy enhancers. This is how you come up with the currency to power your ideal 100-Year Lifestyle.

CHAPTER 4
MASTERING AND MAXIMIZING YOUR PERSONAL ENERGY

The energy drainers and energy enhancers that are a part of your personality and everyday life make up your Dominant Energy Patterns (DEPs). These patterns can be conscious or unconscious. Become aware of them and you can train yourself to shift into a higher gear in an instant.

If you are content with your current energy level and you can see 100 years of exciting living ahead of you, then congratulations. The rest of this book will give you the tools and resources you need to make the most of your solid foundation. If not, you can choose to change your patterns and redefine yourself by identifying your current DEP and consciously choosing a new one, one that will support your 100-Year Lifestyle.

In the movie *Super Size Me*, Morgan Spurlock went from a health nut to fast-food junkie for 30 days to see how this shift in eating patterns would affect his life. He also stopped exercising. Prior to his experiment, he was perfectly healthy and it was amazing what 30 days of fast-food living did to him. His weight ballooned, his cholesterol zoomed, and his liver was showing signs of distress. We should thank Morgan for showing us what happens when you alter your patterns: you alter your life. Morgan also demonstrated that when you change your patterns back, your body heals and becomes healthy again. In other words, like it or not, you become your patterns.

What are your patterns? Really think about it. Your patterns include what you eat, where you shop, what you watch on TV, who you hang around with, the books you read, and more. As a society, we label people by their patterns. We admire "workaholics" and abhor "losers." Some of us are "night owls" and others are "morning persons." We've been on dates with "party animals," "bookworms," and "geeks." We size up other people by their patterns, but rarely do we do so with ourselves.

You can measure your day-to-day connection with your true potential by the intensity of your energy level. Having sustained high energy throughout the day is usually a pretty good indicator that you are operating at your highest level of human potential and your pattern probably supports this. It means you have succeeded in keeping the drama out of your day, avoided second-guessing yourself, and interacted with others from a place of personal integrity. This fuels each hour with purpose. Just the opposite is true if you find yourself constantly scrambling to get by. You can, through the three life-changing principles, permanently re-create your DEP to fuel the rest of your life.

There are five Dominant Energy Patterns (DEPs) that color the outcome of our lives.

1. Destructive patterns
2. Survival patterns
3. Complacency patterns
4. Comfort patterns
5. Human potential patterns

The following are the five Dominant Energy Patterns that shape your life—whether you are aware of it or not. Do you know which pattern colors your life?

DEP #1
DESTRUCTIVE PATTERNS

If you're stuck in a destructive energy pattern, you are probably overspending, overeating, overdrinking, overmedicating, overworking, oversleeping, or overdoing something. You know what it is. Destructive patterns are dangerous because they often end up in addictions or feelings that your life is out of control. It is a pattern usually comprised of repeated behaviors that unconsciously destroy your quality of life.

Maybe the first time you chose the actions related to these patterns, you thought about it before you did it. For instance, the first bite of sugar might have been conscious, but the second, fifth, and tenth were not. Now these patterns occur so spontaneously that you don't even think about them anymore. We all feel better after we buy something, but if you hate yourself after the bill comes because you don't have enough money to pay it, it has become a destructive pattern. If you chose to take the action of this energy pattern consciously right now, would it be your first, second, or even third choice? If not, this may be a destructive pattern for you.

Rather than fueling your human potential, these actions typically leave you empty inside. Some people who are living in a chronic destructive energy pattern can even point to a place on their body where they feel like an "empty well" exists. It may be a hollow pressure in the chest or some other physical manifestation of the emotional pain and emptiness caused by long-term destructive energy patterns.

I believe we all feel this hole in our lives and feel it intensely at one time or another. It is a hole that we want to close but often don't know how. Destructive energy patterns may give you a spike of energy in the beginning, but usually, they are followed by an energy crash filled with anger, resentment, or low self-esteem. They widen the opening rather than closing it to make the pain go away.

It is a bottomless pit that gets larger when it is fed with destructive patterns such as smoking, drinking, drugs, laziness, procrastination, overeating, and erroneous thinking. It also feeds on negative emotions like anger, hopelessness, and hate. How do you reverse the process if you have already arrived at a place where you feel empty, blank, or lost as a result of your choices that are destructive to your long-term well-being? How do you close the hole and refocus your energy? The hole shrinks as you speak and live your truth. It will shrink as you align your actions with your highest vision of yourself one choice at a time, as with Life Changing Principle #2: Change happens one choice at a time. Think progress, not perfection. Every time you make a choice that leads to progress, the hole will feel a little smaller. When you don't, you may get a temporary high followed by a widening of the hole and an empty, hollow feeling inside.

Destructive patterns involve compromising your human potential and not keeping your commitments to yourself. On both a subconscious and a conscious level, your body knows and you know what level of destruction you are causing. Don't ignore the evidence, which causes you to wake up to a much bigger problem down the road.

Destructive energy patterns can be seen in eating, drinking, working, spending, relationships, and more. Here are a few examples:

- Destructive eating patterns can be characterized by automatic or emotional eating and a failure to taste your food when you eat it. You should eat to fuel your body. And you should enjoy your food while you are eating it. Don't eat food out of habit or to alleviate stress.
- Destructive eating patterns also include eating foods that you know are not good for you. Good nutrition is one of our most powerful tools to promote wellness and increase your energy. Healthy eating patterns include reading about and eating foods that promote good health.
- Also, the Blackberry may be the latest e-mail technology craze, but they are not the new blueberries. You should not be plugged into technology around the clock. You have a destructive work pattern when you become stressed by not having immediate access to e-mail, a cell phone, or a computer. You feel that you must be doing something professionally, all the time, and you push the rest of your life away. You are in this pattern if your family and friends frequently refer to you as a workaholic. This type of pattern can take a toll—not only on your health but also on your most important relationships.

- You have destructive relationship patterns when you attract relationships that are controlling, empty, or abusive. Healthy relationships have a good balance of giving and receiving. They nurture you, make you happy, and give you a sense of support. They meet your social and emotional needs.
- Destructive relationship patterns are built more around the "promise" of what may be one day. They tend to feel like work. You can discern the difference between productive and destructive relationships by how you feel after spending time with someone. A sign of emotional maturity is reading (and trusting) the "tea leaves"—your feelings—and avoiding people and situations that will inflict pain. If you must be around these people, just don't give them your energy.

The way out of destructive patterns is to *stop* doing them. Catch yourself in the middle. Become aware of the destructive pattern when it is happening and substitute a new human potential pattern in its place.

DEP #2
SURVIVAL PATTERNS

If you're stuck in a survival pattern, everything is a struggle—from paying your bills to getting to work on time. You always seem to be just one step ahead of disaster. Somehow, however, you generally get by—but without a penny or a second to spare. When you live this type of life, you are fueled by adrenaline. You use stress to get things done. Some people are even addicted to stress. After all, it's a rush. Generally, it makes you feel very important—for a little while. For some people, it even speeds up their metabolisms.

You are in a survival pattern when stress has become normal to you. In fact, when you step back and observe your behavior, you'll find that you actually seek out more stressful experiences. You are late to the meeting—again. You tend to procrastinate and use imminent deadlines to get you motivated. You may even near the limits on your credit cards and be constantly wondering

whether your card will be declined. You live right on the edge—
all the time. You need the rush. People caught up in survival
patterns sometimes refer to themselves as "tornadoes" and the
like—they are whirling masses of energy.

Centenarian Secret   Although living with constant stress is common in today's world, this is not a way to live a sensational century. You might not even make it to 60 or 70. Eventually the roller
coaster catches up to you and the chronic stress has a myriad of
negative consequences. For one thing, it can eventually cause you
to "crash." It's bad for your looks. And longevity experts have now
shown that this chronic stress can shorten your life and precipitate
obesity.

People caught up in survival patterns are generally well inten-
tioned but shortsighted. They struggle to prioritize and figure out
what really matters. Every ounce of energy is spent simply trying
to avoid disaster. For example, when a person's physical or financial health is out of balance, it dominates the expenditure of time
and money. Priorities like buying a spouse a gift, traveling to see
family, or planning a vacation take a back seat.

The good news is that if you are currently in a survival pattern, your commitment to healing will positively impact every
area of your life. To escape a survival pattern, you must *stop* and
realize what you are doing. Catch yourself in the middle, become
aware, and make an energy-enhancing choice. You must learn to
take time-outs and view the bigger picture, build your reserves,
and break the cycle. In some cases, you must reset your internal
barometer and establish a new human potential pattern.

If a stressful job or relationship has moved you into this pattern, you must decide if it is worth it. Living a life in constant
disarray is not a way to thrive or grow. Once you have removed
the stressor, you can change your thinking. Plan long-term, set
boundaries, and avoid constantly putting yourself into situations that will cause you more stress. Focus on building back
your reserves and stop the crisis motivation. To escape a survival

pattern, you need to take control of your life by making different choices that support the vision of your ideal 100-Year Lifestyle, keeping in mind Change Principle #3. Make your future so compelling that you are willing, with each choice in the present, to shift gears midstream.

DEP #3
COMPLACENCY PATTERNS

You've got things together and are getting by without worrying about survival. In a complacency pattern, life isn't a struggle, but it's nothing to write home about either. In this pattern, there is an underlying sense of boredom and laziness. There is no passion. You've resigned yourself to a life of mediocrity.

There is nothing wrong with complacency on occasion. However as a lifestyle, it is boring and will eventually erode your self-esteem and personal confidence. Before you know it, you look in the mirror with disappointment, wondering what ever happened to the flame. The truth is, you can't be mediocre and enjoy a sensational century at the same time. You have to choose. You have resigned yourself to the ho-hum way of life. Do you really want the next 30 to 50 years to stay on this path? It's one thing to be complacent for a week, but for the rest of your life?

Many people in middle age become complacent because they don't believe their efforts will matter. They feel like they have already accomplished what they can and there is not enough time left for them to start a new career, relationship, improve their health, or accumulate money. This pattern will hit home for you if on some level you have given up on your goals. Your actions have no purpose. It's a pattern synonymous with settling, and a why-bother kind of attitude. One of the many challenges of complacency is that you tend to get out of balance with giving and receiving in your relationships.

I've worked with many patients who passionately looked forward to retiring so they could play golf all the time. Once they retired, however, they played so much golf that they didn't enjoy the game anymore. One woman in particular got so bored and disgusted with the game that a year after retiring she sold her clubs and went back to work.

There's no passion with complacency. It can make you feel tired and look older than you actually are. Setting new goals and taking action on them will energize you. Now that you realize you will probably have more time to accomplish all that you've wanted to achieve, why not step things up a notch and embrace your 100-Year Lifestyle? Begin to set some new goals for yourself and start to make them happen. After all, knowing that you may live longer than you ever thought will enable you to start fresh with a lifetime of experience under your belt. Get back in the game:

- If you have grown complacent at work, get back in the game. Start making things happen. Make sure that your superiors recognize your contribution. Instead of saying, "It was nothing" when you are complimented on a project, say, "Thank you for recognizing my role. It was a challenge to bring all the departments together to execute a successful program. But it was very rewarding and I'm very happy to contribute."
- Then, document your achievements. You may even ask your boss to make note of your most recent achievements in a weekly report to his supervisor. Don't go crazy with this, but recognize it for the effective tool that it is. Know that we are now living in a free-agent nation. You must manage your career on a daily basis and build upon your wins. Utilize your documented achievements at annual reviews to ask for a pay raise. Discuss your achievements over the past year with a focus on your results. Show your value to your employer's bottom line.
- When you begin to see positive movement and recognition in your professional life, you will grow less complacent at work.
- If you are in your own business, step up your game, redefine your goals, and take things to the next level.
- If you are retired and are bored out of your mind, commit to a new project, get involved somewhere that you have passion, and engage in life again.

- If you have grown complacent in your personal life, consider taking up a new sport or hobby. What have you always wanted to do? Rediscover an old passion. Maybe you liked to go boating as a kid. Boating can get you out in the sunshine, and the rhythmic feeling of water underneath you lulls you into an almost meditative state. You are one with your surroundings Change things up and take on any type of new activity that is invigorating to you. Choose something, anything, that brings the passion back.

In summary, you escape complacency patterns by setting new goals for yourself and following through on them. You are invigorated by a variety of new experiences that stimulate your mind and by results that show you are still effective in the world. You discover that you can still explore new horizons, whether they are personal or professional. When my children were young, I was unable to go snow skiing as often as I liked. Living in Atlanta, far from the mountains, it seemed like too much of a burden to make an exciting ski trip happen. As my kids grew up, I made the commitment and took the initiative to take everyone on an incredible family ski vacation at least once a year. Everyone got into it and now we all look forward to going. Over the last six years, we have taken some amazing ski vacations together. It is always one of the highlights of our year and it is something we look forward to enjoying for the rest of our lives. Now I am not complacent about my play time anymore. The passion is back and at a higher level than ever.

You will know you are escaping a complacency pattern when you start to feel like a kid again—a kid with a new toy. You are excited and passionate about your extended life.

DEP #4
COMFORT PATTERNS

Life is good. You've worked hard, and you are successful—both professionally and personally. You respect yourself and are surrounded by good people. You've got good habits and a routine that works. But, could it be that your level of comfort is also creating some dis-ease? Deep down, do you think there is more that you would love to experience? Are you worried about rocking the boat?

When you are in a comfort pattern, you are all about maintaining the status quo. You revel in past successes. Unlike the fiery perseverance that got you to where you are today, now you want to avoid making waves. You are generally no longer striving. You feel your days of hard work are behind you—but so is the pleasure of challenging yourself and being in the game. The tire around your waist and hips is starting to expand as your comfort throws you out of balance.

The challenge of a comfort pattern is that it is easy to go from being on a roll to getting in a rut. You generally stop living up to your potential and it is easy to lose your edge.

You often come across people like this in a professional capacity. One example is the doctor who has a good reputation in the community, but suddenly he or she stops investing in the latest techniques and technologies to help patients. You also see this with politicians who strive to get into office by focusing on the needs of the people, and then lose their connection with their constituency. Indeed, when most people look back on their lives, the best times often happen during their "up and coming" years. Too much comfort can really set your life out of balance. Keep that edge. Always look for new ways to make a contribution and use your talents to make a difference. The 100-Year Lifestyle is about achieving the ultimate balance and enjoying that balance for a lifetime.

One character I have always loved is Pigpen from the Peanuts cartoons. Pigpen has a cloud of dirt that surrounds him wherever he goes. When he is moving, the cloud lags behind him. When he stops moving, the cloud of dust catches up to him and gets in his mouth, eyes, and nose. If you are used to being an achiever and you slow down, be on the lookout for the clouds of negativity, boredom, and pessimism that can often come from settling into a comfort pattern. This is often the case when someone retires.

The challenge and opportunity of comfort is to reconnect with a sense of purpose that inspires you while balancing yourself with as much play time as you want. Be careful not to let the comfort become so comfortable that it leads to complacency. When you get stuck in this pattern, you can lose your creativity, sabotage your relationships, or become negative.

Centenarian Secret   You will be truly happy and passionate when you are fully engaged in life again. Not as a robot, doing things the way you always have in the past, but by embracing your life consciously based on what you know you love to do, your worldliness, and experience. Start thinking "outside the box" again for this next phase of your life.

Build spontaneity into your life by the way you choose to spend your time, the places you go, and the people with whom you choose to spend your time. Pursue the projects, innovation, travel, and time with your kids you dream about. Get out of your comfort zone and don't let the dust settle. Your 100-Year Lifestyle is just waiting for you to fan its flames. Use your talents and learn new skills. Enjoy and explore the global playground that is about to be yours as a result of your commitment to your 100-Year Lifestyle.

DEP #5
THE HUMAN POTENTIAL PATTERN: THE SECRET TO A SENSATIONAL CENTURY

In this pattern, you're energized almost all the time. You've got good health, habits, and relationships. You're giving as much or more than you are receiving. You invite change. Your actions are aligned with your life's purpose. You have a pattern of thoughts and actions that consciously support your highest values and human potential.

How do you make your human potential pattern a habit? It begins with your first thought of the day, your first action, your

LIVING THE 100-YEAR LIFESTYLE:
WEIGHT LOSS AND THE 100-YEAR LIFESTYLE

I know about these patterns because, to some degree, I have lived them all—as we all have. In my own life, when I grew comfortable, I also grew fat. I gained close to 40 pounds. I remember preparing a video for my son's thirteenth birthday and looking at myself on the video thinking, *Who is that whale wearing my bathing suit?* My first thought was to lose weight. But there was something about the thought of having a primary goal of *losing* that did not work for me. I had never wanted to "lose" anything, or "lose" at anything before in my life. I never wanted to lose a game of sports, I never wanted to lose anything valuable, and I never wanted to lose in business. I always wanted to win.

I was always one of those people who was motivated by quality of life. I decided that while the extra weight was going to come off my body, it wasn't mine to begin with. It was just an extra burden that I was carrying around that it was time to unload. I decided to develop a new relationship with my abdomen and say goodbye to the extra burden while welcoming all the exciting things that I was going to gain by my commitment to my own human potential pattern. I started saying no to all the foods that tasted good for 30 seconds but were bad for me. I got my "edge" by calling them liars when they would talk to me and tell me to eat them. I started making food and exercise choices that supported my ideal 100-Year Lifestyle. I started focusing on all the things I was gaining, including more energy, feeling younger, being more active, sleeping better, breathing better, looking younger and healthier, and feeling like a kid again. My desire for quality of life kept the feelings of being deprived away that many people who are trying to lose weight often experience. Occasionally I got off track and then got back on track with my next choice (Change Principle #2), knowing that the desire for quality of life gives me lasting motivation and a sense of winning that is greater than the 30 seconds of sweetness that might be provided from sugar. Four years later, I have kept the extra 40 pounds from finding their way back to my body and am practicing and living my ideal 100-Year Lifestyle. I know what you may be going through. If I can do it, you can too.

first everything. You will find that your day goes much better when you start it out in this pattern. Here's a sample scenario where every choice is conscious and builds on the next.

First Thought:
It's good to be alive. I am healing today. I have energy. I am able to manifest abundance in my life through my work and my relationships.

First Action:
Stretch, feel your entire body, breathe deeply, pray, and connect to your goals.

First Feeling:
Experience gratitude, excitement, passion, and hope.

Your energy will dramatically increase when you make your human potential pattern your lifestyle. You will become so energized that even your play time will be filled with more energy. You will need less sleep, less food, and enjoy more of what life has to offer.

DIRECTING YOUR NEW-FOUND ENERGY INTO YOUR 100-YEAR LIFESTYLE

After Lance Armstrong won his seventh Tour de France, one of the announcers commented on how it took cancer to change him. Armstrong said it gave him emotional maturity. He wrote in his book, *It's Not About the Bike*, "If there is a purpose to the suffering that is cancer, I think it must be this: it's meant to improve us." You have an opportunity to redistribute your energy now because you want to, not because your life depends on it. Your old dominant energy patterns can be consciously broken.

Who you will become in the next phase of your life is a direct reflection of how you choose to distribute your energy. You can begin by monitoring your energy and your attitude and shifting toward your human potential.

Have a 100 Percent Conscious Day

Try this today. From the time you wake up in the morning, until the time you go to bed at night, be aware of every moment. Become fully aware of your environment, your emotions, and your activities. You may find that some of who you are and what you do is unconscious, out of control, and not what you would choose for the rest of your life. Some of these things can be changed immediately. If you find yourself trying to control others, or being controlled by others, stop it. Learn to approach your relationships from a place of acceptance, love, and kindness. Make it a policy to only pursue relationships with people who share those same values. Have the same attitude about other behaviors like eating and drinking. If you eat or drink unconsciously, stop before this becomes an addiction. Food and drink are among the great pleasures of life. You deserve to enjoy them, as you would any other relationship—from a place of appreciation, respect, and balance.

Increase Energy Awareness Using Your Breath

One way to increase your awareness of your dominant energy pattern is to monitor your breathing, which is a great indicator of how you are consciously or unconsciously directing your energy. To do this, take a deep breath and feel the full range of motion with your lungs. Go ahead and take another deep breath right now. When we get overwhelmed, our breathing gets shallow and our chest gets tight and rigid around our lungs. Tune into your breathing throughout the day. See if you can catch yourself when you are taking shallow breaths and immediately take some deep ones. Paying attention to the full range of motion in your lungs can immediately bring you to a state of awareness, stop a destructive pattern in its tracks, and give you an opportunity to choose a new pattern.

Increase Energy Awareness Using Your Heart Rate

Monitoring your heart rate is also a great way to become conscious of your dominant energy patterns and how they are affecting your body. Wear a heart monitor, and as you go throughout your day, check your heart rate every 30 minutes. Take note of what causes your heart rate to go up and down. When you feel your intensity rising, look at your heart rate. See if it's rising. If it is, take a deep breath and let the tension out of your body. You will see your heart rate drop back down again. This is a great way to become aware of your unconscious patterns and how they affect you, and immediately gain control over them. When people survive a heart attack, the crisis motivates them to exercise with a heart monitor. Why not do this now as a way to improve your quality of life?

Increase Energy Awareness Using Posture

Your posture is another great way to catch yourself in a pattern that is less than ideal. Do you ever find yourself slouching at your computer, while you are talking on the phone, watching television, or eating a meal? When I mention posture in my seminars it is amazing how instantaneously everyone all of a sudden straightens up. You should tune into your posture regularly throughout the day and when you catch yourself slouching, shift your posture immediately. Train yourself to sit and stand erect. This opens your lungs, is good for your spine, and makes you more confident. Chronic slouching or discomfort when you are erect is a sign that your spine may be out of alignment and balance. I used to see this in my practice all the time and this can easily be corrected with proper care.

CHANGE YOUR PATTERN, CHANGE YOUR LIFE

Like the clothes in your wardrobe, you may wear one energy pattern 20 percent of the time and another 80 percent. Notice what pattern you are in most of the time. Does it suit your current goals? Is it moving you quickly or slowly toward them? Is there another route you would rather take? If so, then change course. Change your posture, breathing, and relax your heart. Take a different action. Choose your new human potential pattern with your ideal 100-Year Lifestyle in mind.

STAY HIGH

Here are some additional tips to help you switch into and sustain high energy to fuel your 100-Year Lifestyle. I'm not talking about hyperactive energy. What I'm talking about is a focused, calm, naturally high state of energy that comes from an inner awareness of your own human potential. You can power your 100-Year Lifestyle:

- By eating high-energy foods:
  o Whole grains
  o Fresh fruits and vegetables
  o Lean meats, fish, and poultry
  o Vegetable proteins
  o Tofu, edamame, flaxseeds, and flaxseed oil
  o High-quality vitamin and mineral supplements
- By engaging in high-energy activities:
  o Fun exercise
  o Getting six to eight hours of restful sleep each night
  o Meaningful work
  o Quality time with family and friends
  o Volunteerism and community service
  o Yoga, PowerCentering, and Pilates
  o Getting a new pet
  o Change-of-pace activities like holding a staff meeting outside, going on a walk with neighbors, taking up a new sport like skiing, cycling, swimming, or boating
- By maintaining high-energy thoughts and attitudes:
  o I accept my current situation and circumstances
  o I have faith that everything will work out
  o I have what it takes to reach my goals
  o I am making a fresh start every day
  o I can choose my pattern at any time
  o I can get off track and get back on track with my next choice
  o I am learning every day
  o I am grateful for all my experiences
  o My challenges teach me the lessons I need to learn

Of course, it's not enough to choose high-energy food, activities, and thoughts. You must also avoid energy drainers such as:

- Eating low-energy foods:
  ○ Processed foods
  ○ Fast foods
  ○ Junk foods
  ○ Sugary desserts
  ○ Foods made with white flour or sugar
  ○ Fried foods
- Engaging in low-energy activities:
  ○ Channel surfing or mindless Web surfing
  ○ Difficult, dull, or stressful work
  ○ Investing time in meaningless relationships
  ○ Overspending
  ○ Falling into a boring routine and losing touch with the fun of life
  ○ Arguing
- Getting caught up on low-energy thoughts and actions:
  ○ I don't accept my current situation and circumstances.
  ○ I don't have faith.
  ○ I don't have what it takes to reach my goals.
  ○ I can't make a fresh start every day.
  ○ I can't choose my pattern at any time.
  ○ I can't get off track and get back on track with my next choice.
  ○ I am not learning every day.
  ○ I am not grateful for all my experiences.
  ○ My challenges don't teach me the lessons I need to learn.
  ○ Why bother?
  ○ I am a victim.

Imagine the Possibility

You've done an amazing job of opening your mind to the possibilities of change. By committing to a potential century or more of life, you are choosing your genetic potential. You are deciding what you want to experience, what condition you want to be in, and what will top your list of achievements along the way. Living a 100-Year Lifestyle will optimize your health, life, love, and relationships as you establish a powerful legacy to live long and strong.

As you find the energy to change, don't worry if things aren't different overnight. Just know that you will get there and your new high-energy human potential pattern will drive the process to your ideal 100-Year Lifestyle.

DISCOVER YOUR POTENTIAL
ACTION PLAN FOR LASTING CHANGE

1. *Take your personal energy inventory and become aware of all of the places that you let your energy leak out into the atmosphere.*
   Choose energy-enhancing thoughts, actions, and feelings and begin to make them a part of who you are.

2. *Decide which Dominant Energy Pattern you are in and begin to identify your personal human potential pattern.*
   Begin making choices following the Three Life-Changing Principles that support your ideal 100-Year Lifestyle where you are living at your best every day.

3. *Have a 100 percent conscious day.*
   Take it all in and be honest with yourself about when you are destructive, complacent, comfortable, and your best. Begin to let go of the things about you that are destructive and rewire yourself for the rest of your 100 years.

4. *Choose energy-enhancing first thoughts, actions, and feelings and reinforce them throughout the day*

5. *Monitor your breathing, heart rate, and posture.*
   Begin with your breathing and posture immediately because they do not require any equipment. When you are ready, invest in a heart monitor and tune into your heart rate. You will be amazed what you learn about yourself during this process.

6. *Choose high-energy foods and activities.*
   When given the choice of low-energy foods and activities, choose high energy. Choose a power walk over being a couch potato. Choose high-energy foods over low-energy foods. Choose healthy interactions with other people rather than destructive interactions.

7. *Stop and choose.*
   When you catch yourself unconsciously doing things that you know you want to change, shift your energy. Literally say to yourself *stop* and physically and emotionally stop yourself. Now make a new choice that supports your ideal 100-Year Lifestyle. Initially you may feel like a tennis ball bouncing back and forth 100 times a day. Eventually you will settle into your human potential pattern, and it will be your lifestyle. You will love it.

PART 3

The Commonsense Strategy of the 100-Year Lifestyle!

We all have a history. I don't want yours and you don't want mine. What's more important than your history is your commitment.

CHAPTER 5
STOP KILLING YOURSELF!

If you want to live an active, healthy, quality life for 100 years and beyond, there is absolutely, positively one thing you are going to have to do. Do you know what that one thing is? Are you ready for this one? This is profound, yet simple—both at the same time. You are going to have to not die. So . . .

STOP KILLING YOURSELF!

There are so many ways that we kill ourselves both quickly and slowly, every day, taking years off our lives and life out of our years. We do this through the small and seemingly insignificant decisions that we make that enhance or detract from our quality of life. We eat the extra cookie, even though we might not even taste it. We skip our evening workout because we are tired, even though we know the workout will energize us. We slump over keyboards all day without moving around and stretching out our legs. What's wrong with this? The problem is that many of us do these things every day—often with the intention of turning over a new leaf. But it's not the resolutions that matter, it's the actions we take every day. It's those very destructive actions or inactions, done over time, that are literally killing us slowly over time. Understand that we have the potential to live a quality 100 years. But many of us will never realize this potential.

The real issue that the 100-Year Lifestyle tackles is not actually when we die or what we die from, but how we live and the choices that we make while we are living. We've all heard a story of a woman or a man who exercised regularly, ate the right foods, goes out for a jog one day and drops dead of a heart attack. While this is certainly sad and shocking, it is also rare. Jogging is not one of the leading causes of death in this country or any other country. This is not a good excuse to continue down a path of self destruction. Many of us justify our poor choices, day in and day out, with stories like this one. We use them as justification for destructive patterns of self-abuse and we use them to build a case against ourselves for why we can't change.

> **Centenarian Secret** There are now around 450 people living who are 110-plus years of age. None of them planned to live this long. They just never died.

One of my patients was a money manager for a large investment-banking firm. He would come to my office for back pain that had been progressing over the years. He was completely out of shape and nearly every organ in his body was unhealthy and not functioning properly. He struggled getting his extra 40 pounds on and off the adjusting table. He came to see me two to three times per year because we were able to put out his fires. We were able to calm the crisis. A wellness adjustment plan was not even in his consciousness even though his family was fully engaged in such a plan and enjoying the benefits of a healthy lifestyle. Preventative health care was like a foreign language to him. Unfortunately, no matter how hard I tried to convince him that he was headed for more serious trouble if he didn't change his lifestyle, he wouldn't listen. When I asked him why he wasn't willing to be more proactive about his health, he told me the story about the jogger. What a ridiculous excuse to perpetuate his suffering. He would only make his health a priority when his suffering—crisis motivation—kicked in at its highest level.

Living the 100-Year Lifestyle is not simply about not dying; it is about the quality of your life. Nobody I have ever met has driven by a nursing home and said, "That's where I'd like to end up." We don't just "end up" in there; we kill ourselves slowly over time. This man was suffering on so many levels because of his lack of commitment to a 100-Year Lifestyle. He would say things like, "I want to just live for today" and "I just want to enjoy my life." But what's enjoyable about feeling like you're going to pass out every time you walk up a flight of stairs? What's enjoyable about working yourself into the ground without enjoying good times with your family and friends along the way? Every choice you make to produce a quality 100-Year Lifestyle will also improve the quality of your life today.

I was recently flying back from Philadelphia after giving a keynote speech to a group of health care providers, and I sat next to a musician who was coming back from a gig. We talked about his music career and his family for a while. He was about 100 pounds overweight and not taking care of his body at all. His diet consisted completely of junk food. He told me that he ate too much and drank too much. As our discussion progressed he asked me what I did for a living. I told him that I was a chiropractor and a professional speaker. I told him about this book. He told me that he knew that he needed to make changes in his life, and he already knew what they were. He said his unhealthy lifestyle was causing tremendous suffering. He had shortness of breath, back and neck pain, fatigue, and excessive stress—not to mention the strain on his heart was too much to bear.

He then told me about his 98-year-old grandfather, who was still in good health and enjoying life. He realized he had the same genetic potential as his grandfather, but he also knew that he had to take responsibility and *stop killing himself* today, or he wasn't going to come close to fulfilling his longevity potential. Shortly before we departed, he told me that he was going to start making some "serious changes now." Otherwise, he said, he wasn't going to make it. I told him I wished him well. He had an exciting road ahead. The resolution he made that day was easy. All the little choices he would make from that day forward would determine his success or failure down the road. Three months later I called to see how he was doing and he was thrilled. He told me that he had begun to make the changes that would get him back on track. He had lost 15 pounds, replaced the post-gig midnight eating and drinking binges with a power walk, and he had started seeing a chiropractor to take care of his spine. He was excited about the possibility of living a healthy 100 years. He said to me passionately, "I've got a lot of music in me."

We'll take a look, in the next chapter, at the leading causes of death in this country. You will see that the causes here are not the leading causes of death in all countries. You will also see that the majority of these conditions are preventable if you are willing to live a healthy lifestyle. As you look at the list you may find yourself making a comment like "that's what my father died from." You may even say, "My grandparents died from that," and "This disease runs in my family."

Even though our parents and grandparents may have passed away from diseases with a genetic component to them, your

▶ **LIVE LONG AND STRONG EXERCISE**
STOP KILLING YOURSELF

Effective immediately, I will stop killing myself by eliminating the following habits that I know are not good for me.

_____

_____

_____

_____

_____

_____

_____

_____

_____

parents probably outlived your grandparents by a good 5, 10, 20, or even 30 years. The important thing to remember is, for most of us, we not only inherited a set of genes, but we inherited a way of thinking and living as well—a lifestyle. In our generation, for example, we see a lot of stressed-out parents—"hyper-parents"— struggling to balance work and kids. Times have changed, but instead of realigning our values, we just paddle harder. Most of us are now in debt and stressed about money. Our unwillingness to change with changing times keeps us in survival and destructive energy patterns that take years off of our life, and life from our years. Think of someone trying to dance to disco even after the music has changed to rap. You would see a whirlwind of activity, in all the wrong directions. This is what happens when we resist change—the toll it takes on our minds, bodies, and spirits can be very damaging. This leads to a 60-, 70- or 80-Year Lifestyle versus the active, healthy 100-Year Lifestyle we deserve.

Centenarian Secret　Only around half of centenarians have had first-degree relatives or grandparents who also achieved very old age. Many have exceptionally old siblings.

The average life expectancy for men, currently, is just 74 or 75 years. The average life expectancy for women, currently, is just 79 or 80 years. Average means that some people are living much longer, and some people are dying much younger. Where will you fall? What will your quality of life be along the way? The health choices you make today will absolutely impact your quality of life now and in the future.

You are designed to thrive under changing circumstances. But you must first listen to your body's innate wisdom. You must learn self-trust—a vital component of the 100-Year Lifestyle. After all, life is a series of transitions, and the one you are about to go on—embracing the reality of your potential longevity—can be the most exciting time of your life. Confront the unknown with the knowledge that on the other side of letting go is a tremendous feeling of freedom, youthfulness, and renewal. This is where you will thrive. Remember Change Principle #1: Change is easy. Thinking about change is hard.

LISTEN TO YOUR BODY'S INNATE INTELLIGENCE

Your mind, body, and spirit are amazing. They are driven to thrive by an innate intelligence, an inner wisdom that makes approximately 8,000,000 new blood cells in your bone marrow every second. Your bones are constantly rebuilding themselves

▶ **BABY STEPS TO A BABY CLOTHES BONANZA**

Consider Leda McIntosh Jackson, who started Pixie Lily in the late 1990s. Today, her layettes are in 500 stores around the country and are must-haves among many celebrities. But nine years ago, she simply had a good idea and no idea how to make it work. After all, she was also the mother of a newborn. And she wanted to make handcrafted, vintage-inspired baby clothes, using fine fabrics and details like crochet and embroidery.

She began by taking orders on a small scale and sewing at home while the baby slept. "It was all about baby steps, back then," she says. "I was encouraged to do that—to simply start sewing, testing the waters, figuring things out as I went." The concept caught on and she eventually figured out how to mass-market her concept and make money.

She attributes much of her success to prioritizing. Thinking progress, not perfection is key.

"I feel that we ask so much of mothers these days," she says. "Now you don't just have to bring cupcakes to school; you have to bring homemade cupcakes from scratch with every child's initials done in calligraphy on the frosting. We are all trying to show one another how great we are with managing everything. You just can't. I mean, I've got dust bunnies in my house that are actually going to war. They have divided themselves into tribes. But I really think that you have to prioritize and you have to learn to say 'no' and that's not a very popular thing."

and are not at all static. Your heart beats an average of 60 times per minute, or an incredible 3 billion times over the course of 100 years. Studies have shown that to build your incredible body from scratch would drain all the treasures of the world with no guarantee of success. Why would you kill yourself slowly over time and deteriorate your original parts? It's time to stop killing yourself and start keeping yourself functioning at your highest level. I've made a career of watching people embrace this philosophy and fall in love with their results. You will too.

Your genetic wisdom is trying to assert itself every day, trying to guide you to what is best for you. Did your parents and grandparents test the limits of their genetic potential? Not even close. So, let's not use our family history as a reason to not live the 100-Year Lifestyle we deserve. Instead, let's look at choices that support your longevity and maximize your sensational century. I understand that you may make sacrifices on occasion for the sake of your family or work. Sacrifices are inevitable. But make them from a place of awareness. Choose your sacrifice and live in balance.

Centenarian Secret   "Centenarians disprove the perception that 'the older you get, the sicker you get,' centenarians teach us that the older you get the healthier you've been."—The New England Centenarian Study

As a society, we are very focused on the external. We spend our days striving to achieve external worth, while slowly killing ourselves on the inside. This is a destructive pattern. The decisions that have the greatest impact on your health are not the big ones, like starting a new diet. They are the seemingly insignificant ones you make day to day that perpetuate destructive patterns and kill you slowly over time.

Your genes play a role in your longevity, but a much smaller one than you would think. If you explore the top killers of people in our society today, you'll find that most are preventable through lifestyle choices that are good for you. People have a greater chance of living to be 100 when they stay relatively healthy throughout their lives. As the New England Centenarian Study researchers learned, 90 percent of centenarians have been functionally independent the vast majority of their lives, up until the average age of 92 years.

A smaller percentage of centenarians make it after overcoming a serious illness. But they are the exception and not the rule. For most of these people, crisis motivated them to change. But why not avoid the crisis to begin with? Why put yourself in a position to need a modern-day miracle? There are very few magic bullets. The way you care for yourself, and the environment in which you live, will have the greatest impact on your health and longevity. Patients and colleagues used to tell me all the time, "You are a miracle worker, doc." Wouldn't it be better to keep yourself healthy so you never needed a miracle?

> **Centenarian Secret** Many centenarian women have had children after the age of 35 and even 40 years of age. Having children after 40 may be a sign that a woman's reproductive system is aging slowly—and that the rest of her body is aging slowly as well. Additionally, women who have children after 40 have four times a greater chance of living to 100.

You will be excited to learn that the leading causes of death are all preventable. While you may have some of them in your family history, the commonsense and proven strategies that follow may help you to postpone them for decades or even wipe them out of your future completely.

CHAPTER 6
AVOIDING THE TOP TEN LEADING CAUSES OF PREVENTABLE DEATH

We all know that people die every day. According to the U.S. National Center for Health Statistics, 2,443,387 people died in the year 2002. Of these, 1,199,264 of them were men and 1,244,123 of them were female. The leading causes of death were heart disease, cancer, cerebrovascular diseases like stroke, chronic lower respiratory diseases, Alzheimer's, diabetes, the flu, and pneumonia. If you are like many people, you probably have at least a little concern about at least one of these conditions. For example, your father may have died of a heart attack, and now you fear dying from one as well. Maybe your mother or grandparents suffered from cancer and the thought of you experiencing the same fate is a little scary. Their destiny does not have to be yours.

The charts on the right, created by the Center for Disease Control, give the leading causes of death for all races of both females and males by age group.

These rankings apply to the entire population and all age groups. Take men and heart disease, for example. Although heart disease is the single biggest threat to a man's longevity, it actually surpasses all other causes of death for men between the ages 45 and 54, and then ages 65 and over. From childhood until age 44, accidents are actually the single biggest threat to a man's life.

It's important to understand that disease generally does not jump out of the closet at you. If you are paying attention to your innate intelligence, you will be alerted when something is amiss. Typically, you will experience some sort of physical or mental

Leading Causes of Death for Females—United States, 2002

ALL RACES, FEMALE	PERCENT
Number 1: Heart Disease	28.6
Number 2: Cancer	21.6
Number 3: Stroke	8.0
Number 4: Chronic lower respiratory diseases	5.3
Number 5: Alzheimer's disease	3.4
Number 6: Diabetes	3.1
Number 7: Unintentional injuries	3.0
Number 8: Influenza and pneumonia	3.0
Number 9: Kidney disease	1.7
Number 10: Septicemia	1.5

Leading Causes of Death for Males—United States, 2002

ALL RACES, MALE	PERCENT
Number 1: Heart Disease	28.4
Number 2: Cancer	24.1
Number 3: Unintentional injuries	5.8
Number 4: Stroke	5.2
Number 5: Chronic lower respiratory diseases	5.1
Number 6: Diabetes	2.9
Number 7: Influenza and pneumonia	2.4
Number 8: Suicide	2.1
Number 9: Kidney disease	1.6
Number 10: Chronic liver disease	1.5

disharmony or "dis-ease" before you get sick. Maybe you feel out of balance and fatigue sets in. Your digestion or elimination patterns may change. When you heed the early warning signs, and your body is functioning at its highest level through proactive health and lifestyle strategies, you can often prevent them from occurring in the first place. It makes much more sense to maintain and preserve your body's natural defense system. Too often, we shift into self-care only after we experience symptoms of disease. This is not very effective, as symptoms are often the last sign of a serious problem. This is crisis motivation. In a state of homeostasis, the body fights off disease and infection on its own. It keeps your arteries clean and it eliminates rabid cells that can turn into cancer. Work with your body's natural ability to function properly, keep it in balance, and enjoy a healthy 100 years.

In the following section, we will take a look at the leading causes of death in this country. Again, what's interesting is that these are not the leading causes of death in all countries. We are going to talk about some of the lifestyle and dietary differences in nations around the world and how you might be able to incorporate some of these changes into your own life, today, as part of your 100-Year Lifestyle.

Do you realize the degree of control you have over your health? If you have a genetic disposition to any type of life-threatening condition, fearlessly take the proactive steps to reduce the chance that it will affect your life and live your life to the fullest. This commonsense strategy is exciting and I encourage you to passionately pursue knowledge like this throughout your life.

Centenarian Secret   Pomegranate juice may help reduce cholesterol. Turmeric may help prevent Alzheimer's.

MANAGING YOUR HEALTH TO 100 YEARS AND BEYOND

Let's take a look at preventative measures you can take against the leading causes of death. This information has been condensed here for your easy access and implementation. The solutions that are presented are not a mystery that was just discovered. They are well documented scientifically and are just waiting for you to make them a part of your lifestyle.

Heart Disease

According to the National Health and Nutrition Examination Survey, over 70 million people in this country suffer from one or more form of cardiovascular disease. Sixty million have high blood pressure, and an astounding 80 million have high cholesterol. Heart disease is the leading cause of death for men and women in this country. Men tend to develop it at high percentages sooner than women. This is why it's traditionally considered more of a "male" problem—many men die from it in their prime.

Comparatively, heart disease is not the leading cause of death in places like Okinawa, Japan. Okinawans have 80 percent fewer heart attacks than North Americans. When they have a heart attack, they are twice as likely to survive. However, when they migrate to this country and adopt our lifestyle, they take on our same arterial risk. How much more do you need to know? Take heart. It's largely about choices. Even if you have currently been diagnosed with heart disease, it has been shown that you can help reverse it through diet and lifestyle. Tom Kirk, a certified financial planner in Orlando, Florida, did just that. His incredible story appears on the following page.

There are some obvious ways to prevent heart disease. First, we know that you can reduce your risk of heart disease by not smoking. Maintaining a healthy weight is also key. Pear-shaped figures have less heart disease than "apple-shaped" figures, which are so common among middle-aged men. A diet rich in fruits and vegetables and low in fat is very important. There are tricks you will discover as you learn more about diet. For example, pomegranate juice can, in fact, help reduce your cholesterol, and three grams of Omega-3 fatty acids a day are good for the heart. I encourage you to read everything you can about heart-healthy fitness and nutrition. Living a heart-healthy lifestyle will support you in achieving your 100-Year Lifestyle.

Tom Kirk

"I am a survivor of triple bypass, open-heart surgery that I had at the age of 46. There is no heart disease in my family. I don't smoke or drink, and I am not overweight. I don't have high blood pressure. My total cholesterol was 190.

Through diet, exercise, and the recommendations of my cardiologist, I have made great strides toward living a normal life expectancy. My cardiologist said my case was a good news/bad news story. The good news was that I was only 46 and in otherwise good health when I had my surgery, so I could expect to recover quickly. The bad news was that I was only 46 and had already had major heart surgery. He said that if they do a bypass operation on a 65-year-old and it lasts for 20 years, the patient is 85 and has lived a normal life span. If my surgery lasts 20 years, I will only be 66. So I immediately began exercising three to four times per week, eating only 15 grams of saturated fat a day, eating red meat only twice per year, eggs once per month, avoiding cheese and dairy products, and taking a statin called Pravachol. This resulted in some improvement to my blood chemistry, but not enough. As you may know, the target numbers for heart attack survivors are much lower than for those who have not had a heart attack.

I read that you need to exercise six days per week for at least 45 minutes and that you need to stay away from junk food and manage your portions of food. After six months, my total cholesterol is now 150, my good cholesterol is 45, my bad cholesterol is 90, and my triglycerides are 78. All these numbers are below the low targets set for people like me. My cardiologist said that the exercise routine I was on was having an effect on my blood chemistry equal to and perhaps greater than the medication that I was also taking.

My other risk factor is that I am an overachieving, A-type, adrenalin junkie. This constant state is corrosive to your arteries. Exercise reduces the level of the harmful chemicals in your body by burning them off. Exercise also creates favorable brain chemistry, which is calming. Through reading, yoga, and meditation I am injecting peace and quiet into the chaos. Frankly, this is the hardest thing for me to do in my recovery. Exercising six days per week is a breeze compared to changing the way I look at and respond to the world around me."

Seriously consider exercise, nutrition, and other forms of holistic approaches to change your numbers prior to taking medication. If your doctor does suggest you start a heart medication regimen, always learn about the potential side effects of medications. Also, look for lifestyle changes that you can make to avoid them when possible. Speak to your doctor if you have a family history of heart disease, and develop a plan that will serve your goals for your extended life. If you depend on medication without changing your lifestyle, you will probably be stuck in that regimen for the next 30, 40, or 50 years.

Centenarian Secret   According to the American Heart Association, your total cholesterol should remain below 200 mg/DL. LDL should be below 130 mg/DL. HDL should be 40 mg/DL or higher. Your blood pressure should be below 120/80. Stay up on the latest "normal" numbers, as they will occasionally change, and most important, keep your body functioning at its optimum level with healthy habits.

Here are some other basic guidelines:

- Don't smoke or use other tobacco products.
- Eat a varied diet, rich in fruits, vegetables, and low-fat foods.
- Maintain a healthy weight.
- Consume alcohol in moderation.
- Get at least 30 minutes of aerobic exercise three to five days per week.
- Keep your cholesterol levels in normal ranges.
- Control your blood sugar if you have diabetes.
- Control your blood pressure and cholesterol with diet and exercise before committing to a lifetime of medication.
- Relax. Eliminate physical and emotional stressors.
- Monitor your blood chemistry, heart rate, and blood pressure.
- Visit the American Heart Association Web site to learn more.
- Implement the Health Care Hierarchy of the 100-Year Lifestyle in the next chapter.

Cancer

Cancer is the second leading cause of death for men and women. Lung cancer is the most common type of cancer. Approximately 164,000 Americans are diagnosed each year. Around 87 percent of lung cancer is linked to cigarette smoking. Prostate cancer is also very common. In fact, 80 percent of men over the age of 80 now develop it. Scientists believe that hereditary prostate cancer accounts for just 9 percent of all cases. A high-fat diet is believed to be a contributing factor. Prostate cancer is very rare in places like Okinawa, where the diet tends to be low in fat.

Breast cancer rates are also very rare there, as they are throughout most of Japan. Scientists think that a key factor is the daily consumption of phytoestrogens through natural sources like soy and tofu. In fact, many men with prostate cancer in the United States now make phytoestrogen-rich flaxseed and flaxseed oil a part of their diets. Tomatoes—a rich source of lycopene—also mitigate chances of prostate cancer. I encourage you to read everything you can about nutrition and lifestyle to prevent cancer and keep your body functioning at its highest level. Don't stop with the news. Lifelong learning is a key component of the 100-Year Lifestyle.

Some basic guidelines:

- Don't smoke or use other tobacco products.
- Eat a varied diet, rich in fruits, vegetables, fiber, and low-fat foods. Don't just eat healthy foods out of the fear of getting sick. Eat to enjoy and promote a healthy 100-Year Lifestyle.
- Maintain a healthy weight.
- Get at least 30 minutes of exercise three to five days per week.
- Avoid overexposure to the sun and use sunscreen.
- Drink alcohol only in moderation, if at all.
- Be aware of potential cancer-causing substances (carcinogens) in your home and workplace, and take steps to reduce your exposure to these substances.
- Have regular preventive health screenings.
- Know your family health history and review it with your doctor.

- Visit the American Cancer Society Web site to learn more.
- Implement the Health Care Hierarchy of the 100-Year Lifestyle in the next chapter.

Are you beginning to see that most of these items qualify as commonsense? Avoiding these choices causes dis-ease, disharmony, weakness, and imbalance that stresses your nervous system and heart, and makes you less adaptable to the world around you. Your energy is redistributed and goes toward survival and battling the negative impact of the stress rather than on optimizing your genetic capabilities. Your body's intelligence gets redirected and diverted.

Accidents

Talk about preventable! Accidents are a leading cause of death in this country. In fact, accidents rank third among the leading causes of death for men. Let's wake up! Certainly there are many unavoidable dangers in the world. Things happen. But you have to look no further than a mountain biking trail to see how many men are wired. We love to test our limits, and then some. Although car accidents remain the most pervasive risk for accidental deaths, men are almost twice as likely as women to drive drunk—another avoidable risk. To reduce your chances of a fatal crash:

- Wear your seat belt.
- Keep your speed down.
- Practice defensive driving.
- Don't drive while sleepy or under the influence of drugs or alcohol.

Poisoning is the second leading cause of fatal accidents to men. To reduce your risk of poisoning:

- Place carbon monoxide and smoke detectors near bedrooms in your house.
- Have fuel-burning appliances inspected each year.

- Store household products in their original containers.
- Read and follow label instructions for household products.
- Beware of pill popping. Stop the destructive pattern of popping a pill every time you feel a symptom. Let your body heal itself. If you absolutely have to take medication, make sure you follow label instructions carefully and practice self-care and health care strategies to minimize their need and offset potential side effects.
- Ventilate areas where you use chemical products.
- Post the poison control number, (800) 222-1222, by each telephone in your home, especially if you have children or grandchildren.
- Install air and water filtrations systems in your home and replace the filters regularly.

Falls and drowning are also leading causes of fatal injury. Commonsense precautions include using a safety ladder, placing nonskid mats in showers and tubs, and never swimming alone. Also, many fatal injuries happen at work. So please follow all necessary precautions while on the job. Everyone says, "This can't happen to me." Use common sense. If you say to yourself, "I shouldn't be doing this," don't.

Alzheimer's

Alzheimer's affects approximately one in ten people in this country over the age of 65 and about one in two over the age of 85. However, this isn't the case everywhere. Elderly villagers in India have the lowest rates of Alzheimer's in the world and scientists are starting to suspect why. They think it's connected to their high consumption of curcumin. Curcumin is a compound found in the spice turmeric. Curcumin has powerful antioxidant and anti-inflammatory properties and Indians eat turmeric with most every meal. Animal studies are starting to confirm the connection. Also, older adults whose total folate intake is at or above the recommended daily guidelines can cut their risk of developing Alzheimer's by as much as 50 percent. Folate is found in liver, leafy green vegetables, broccoli, oranges, asparagus, and many other foods.

> **Centenarian Secret**   One-third of centenarians have had no significant changes in their thinking abilities. High homocysteine levels, on the other hand, may contribute to dementia or Alzheimer's. However, homocysteine levels may be reduced by taking folate with vitamins B_6 and B_{12}. You can further reduce your risk of Alzheimer's by maintaining a healthy cardiovascular system. Visit the Alzheimer's Association Web site for more information.

Stroke

Strokes can be debilitating, and they are also preventable. Over time, sufferers often develop symptoms of dementia. A small stroke can also masquerade as dementia. The guidelines for reducing your chances of a stroke are similar to those for heart disease. Work to keep your blood pressure within normal ranges. You can't control some risks, such as family history, age, and race, but you can control the leading cause—high blood pressure—as well as contributing factors such as smoking and diabetes. Follow the diet of populations around the world that tend not to have strokes. This means a low-calorie, plant-based diet that is high in unrefined carbohydrates. Additional preventive measures include:

- Lower your intake of cholesterol and saturated fat.
- Don't smoke.
- Control diabetes.
- Maintain a healthy weight.
- Get at least 30 minutes of exercise three to five days per week.
- Manage stress.
- Limit alcohol consumption.
- Visit the American Stroke Association Web site to learn more.
- Implement the Health Care Hierarchy of the 100-Year Lifestyle in the next chapter.

Chronic Obstructive Pulmonary Disease (COPD)

Chronic obstructive pulmonary disease (COPD) is a group of chronic lung conditions that includes emphysema and chronic bronchitis. Once again, they are also preventable. Such lung conditions makes it more and more difficult to breathe, and breathing is one of those very important functions that you want to excel at for a lifetime. COPD is strongly associated with lung cancer, the leading cause of cancer deaths among men (and women). The main cause is smoking. Studies show that few centenarians have a substantial history of smoking. In fact, very few have ever smoked. Another risk factor is exposure to indoor or outdoor pollutants. Nearly 20 percent of cases are also attributed to work-related exposure.

Some preventive measures you can take:

- Don't smoke.
- Avoid secondhand smoke.
- Minimize exposure to workplace chemicals.
- Use air filters in your home and work to ensure that you breathe the cleanest air possible, especially if you live in a city where smog alerts are common.
- Visit the American Lung Association Web site to learn more.
- Implement the Health Care Hierarchy of the 100-Year Lifestyle in the next chapter.

Pneumonia and influenza are especially life-threatening to people whose lungs have already been damaged by COPD, asthma, or smoking. The risk of death from pneumonia or influenza is also higher among people with heart disease, diabetes, or a weakened immune system due to AIDS or immunosuppressive drugs. You can keep your resistance high with exercise, stress-free living, and a healthy diet, and by keeping your spine, nerve, and immune system functioning properly and breathing clean air.

Diabetes

There are several types of diabetes. All of them can be managed and research shows that type 2 diabetes is also preventable or can be postponed for many years. It results when your body no longer uses insulin correctly. This is the most common form of diabetes. Approximately 18.2 percent of Americans have diabetes and almost one-third of those people don't know they have it. An additional 41 million people have prediabetes—or impaired glucose tolerance.

Excess body fat, especially around the middle, is an important risk factor for diabetes. About 80 percent of people who have the disease are either overweight or obese. The diabetes complications most likely to be fatal are heart disease and stroke, which occur at two to four times the average rate in people with diabetes. People with diabetes haven't benefited as much from recent advances in heart disease treatment as have people without diabetes. During the past 30 years, deaths from heart disease have fallen 36 percent in men without diabetes, as compared with only 13 percent in men who have diabetes. Some preventive measures you can take:

- Maintain a healthy weight.
- Eat a varied diet, rich in fruits, vegetables, and low-fat foods.
- Get at least 30 minutes of exercise three to five days per week.
- Get your fasting blood sugar level checked periodically.
- Know your family's diabetes history and discuss it with your doctor.
- Visit the American Diabetes Association Web site to learn more.
- Implement the Health Care Hierarchy of the 100-Year Lifestyle in the next chapter.

Suicide

In 2002, 25,409 men committed suicide. Men commit suicide four times as often as women do. Depression—which is estimated to affect 7 percent of men in any given year—is an important risk factor for suicide. But male depression may be underdiagnosed, partly because men are less likely than women are to seek treatment for it or perform the proactive self-care or health care strategies for prevention. In addition, men don't always develop standard symptoms such as sadness, feelings of worthlessness, and excessive guilt. Instead, they may be more likely to complain of fatigue, irritability, sleep disturbances, and loss of interest in work or hobbies. Substance abuse—which is more common in men—can mask depression and make it more difficult to diagnose. People at risk of suicide may:

- Be depressed, moody, socially withdrawn, or aggressive
- Have suffered a recent life crisis
- Show changes in personality
- Feel worthless
- Abuse alcohol or drugs
- Have frequent thoughts about death
- Talk about death and self-destruction

If you find yourself avoiding others, feeling hostile and worthless, thinking about death, and using alcohol and drugs to numb your pain, you are in a destructive energy pattern. Shift yourself by changing your Dominant Energy Pattern on your own, or if you need to, with the help of a professional. In an urgent situation, an emergency room or crisis center can help. Friends or family members may be the first to notice your uncharacteristic behavior. Take their advice and seek help.

Kidney Disease

Kidney failure, most often a complication of diabetes or high blood pressure, sends an estimated 400,000 Americans into crisis each year. Control of diabetes and high blood pressure can prevent or slow the progression of kidney disease. Another cause of kidney failure is overuse of medications such as NSAIDS (nonsteroidal anti-inflammatory drugs), such as ibuprofen (Advil, Motrin, etc.) that are toxic to the kidneys. Some preventive measures you can take:

- Drink plenty of fluids.
- Exercise regularly.
- Maintain your proper weight.
- Don't smoke.

- Get checked regularly for diabetes and high blood pressure.
- Make excellent self-care and drug-free health care choices whenever possible to prevent and minimize your need for both prescription and over-the-counter medication.
- Visit the National Kidney Foundation Web site to learn more.
- Implement the Health Care Hierarchy of the 100-Year Lifestyle in the next chapter.

Chronic Liver Disease and Cirrhosis

Cirrhosis is the tenth leading cause of death nationwide, causing approximately 25,000 deaths each year. The leading cause of liver disease, in general, is alcoholism, which takes a heavy toll on men in general. Men account for more than 70 percent of the 75,000 alcohol-attributable deaths that occur each year in the United States.

Other leading causes of chronic liver disease and cirrhosis include hepatitis B and C and certain inherited diseases such as hemochromatosis, in which abnormal amounts of iron accumulate in the liver. Nonalcoholic fatty liver disease, which is associated with obesity, also sometimes leads to cirrhosis. Some preventive measures you can take:

- Don't drink alcohol to excess.
- Take precautions when using possibly hazardous chemicals.
- Practice safe sex.
- Don't inject street drugs.
- Make excellent self-care and drug-free health care choices whenever possible.
- Maintain a healthy weight.
- Visit the American Liver Foundation Web site to learn more.
- Implement the Health Care Hierarchy of the 100-Year Lifestyle in the next chapter.

YOU DESERVE TO BE HEALTHY FOR A LIFETIME

Make your health a priority and keep yourself healthy for a lifetime. Understand the potential risks of your family history, but instead of worrying about them make lifestyle choices today, and every day, to support the quality of your longevity. Trust your body's ability to adapt to your environment and nurture its adaptability through your 100-Year Lifestyle choices. It will improve your life today and tomorrow. Educate yourself. Eat healthy foods, stay physically active, keep your spine and nervous system aligned and balanced, stay away from cigarettes, get regular checkups, and guard against accidents every day. By making this a way of life, you'll increase your chances of staying healthy and active beyond 100 years, or for however many years you have left.

▶ WRITE A NEW FAMILY TREE

Gather health data on all of your immediate family members. For any members who have passed away, find out what they died from.

Your mother: _____

Your father: _____

Your father's parents: _____

Your mother's parents: _____

Your siblings: _____

TURN OVER A NEW LEAF:

Since I have a family history of _____, _____, and _____, the healthy habits that I will begin immediately are:

1. _____

2. _____

3. _____

4. _____

5. _____

Remember Change Principle Number 2: Change comes one choice at a time. Think progress, not perfection. The Titration Principle can impact you negatively just as it can impact you positively. Smoking cigarettes is the most obvious and easy-to-embrace example of this concept. It is not the first cigarette that kills you. It is also not the last cigarette that kills you. It is the cumulative affect of all of the cigarettes over time that damages your lungs. Eventually this overwhelms the coping mechanisms of your body.

Centenarian Secret Titian, the well-known Italian master painter born in the late 1400s, lived to at least 90 years of age. Some reports indicate he lived to 99 years of age! Hippocrates, who was born in 460 B.C., died in his mid-eighties.

The same applies with obesity. Stop killing yourself with food. It is not an extra scoop of ice cream today that puts on the extra pounds. It's the accumulation of all the extra scoops over time. Are a few minutes of pleasure really worth it? Can you find healthier ways to treat yourself? Just like smoking, destructive eating patterns compromise our lives. Eating should always be a conscious choice. Try to make good choices ever day. Remember: Think progress, not perfection. Choose with your ideal 100-Year Lifestyle in mind.

Without becoming another diet book, but understanding the importance of good nutrition, here is some basic eating advice of the 100-Year Lifestyle. If you ever say to yourself, "I shouldn't be eating that," you shouldn't. If your innate intelligence tells you, "I should eat a salad today," you should listen. If your body is telling you it needs more fiber, vegetables, or protein, you should listen to it and give your body what it needs.

Unfortunately, many of our destructive patterns have created confusion in our own minds. We don't know which voice to listen to. Begin to trust yourself again and connect to your inner voice. Healthy thoughts and actions lead to a healthy life and nobody is going to be able to make these choices for you.

It's a step-by-step process, one choice at a time; think progress, not perfection.

Centenarian Secret Lifelong vegetarians visit the hospital 22 percent less often than meat eaters, and have shorter stays. Vegetarians suffer 20 percent less premature mortality from all causes, compared with their meat-eating counterparts, according to the BBC online news service.

As I have traveled around the world, I have spoken to thousands of individuals who have made this shift in thinking. They know that their diet affects how they look and feel. They align their diets to those values. They have the same passion for food as everyone else. But instead of eating bacon with scrambled eggs, they may have wild Alaskan sockeye salmon with an egg-white omelet. Instead of cooking with margarine, they may use cold-pressed extra-virgin olive oil. They have a healthy glow that comes from drinking purified water throughout the day. They are eating with their 100-Year Lifestyle in mind. This benefits their lives today—they look and feel better—and it promotes longevity.

Fueling Your 100-Year Lifestyle

I would like to end this chapter with a short discussion of some superfoods that will help you "fuel" your 100-Year Lifestyle and stay healthy. First of all, some common mistakes: Women need protein and can age faster when they don't get enough of it. Protein is very important to men also. What you want to focus on are healthy protein sources. Always go organic when possible. Although it's more expensive, you'll be glad you did. We will spend more time on this in the next chapter. Consider stocking your refrigerator with an organic chicken. You can cook the chicken and then make it into a light chicken salad for lunch or dinner, seasoning it with a golden onion—organic of course. In terms of mayonnaise, delicious soy-based mayonnaises are now available that taste just as good as the old stuff. Chicken salad makes a satisfying meal, but it is also a wonderful side dish.

Tofu and soy are great sources of protein and can be prepared a variety of ways. Fish is also a great source of protein; however, as we all know, we must be careful with fish. A good selection is wild Alaskan sockeye salmon. Salmon is good for your body and skin. Surprisingly, you can also find good quality salmon in cans at the grocery store. But you want to avoid farmed salmons. Did you know that farmed salmon is actually naturally gray in color?

Some additional superfoods include:

- Wild salmon
- Blueberries
- Broccoli
- Tomatoes
- Soy
- Flaxseed
- Oats
- Strawberries
- Cantaloupe
- Garlic
- Beans
- Green tea

You have to be careful with fruits like strawberries. The best option may actually be to grow them at home since it is difficult to find organic strawberries. Plant a handful of strawberry plants, and they can easily fill up a garden bed in two to three years, with very little care. You will be pleased: nothing compares with the color and taste of a freshly picked, vine-ripened strawberry.

In fact, your best bet in many cases will be to grow your own fruits and vegetables during the warmer months. This is the purest form of organic eating. Easy things to grow include tomatoes, lettuce, cucumbers, and herbs like chives, parsley, and basil. Plant enough basil and you will have a steady supply all summer long of fresh pesto and greens to mix with your salads. In southern climates, chives and parsley keep producing all winter long.

What you can expect, when you eat this way, is a healthy glow and an overall sense of wellness. To the degree you can, try to get a little exercise after each meal. Especially as you age, this really helps your body utilize the nutrients you take in. You can practice true organic gardening by building or mixing garden beds with compost from the nursery. If you are making a garden bed, the mixture is one-third compost, one-third peat moss, and one-third perilite. Organic fertilizers are even available to nourish your soil and help your garden thrive.

TRUST YOUR INNATE INTELLIGENCE

The regenerative powers of your body are amazing. Have faith in it. Support it every day through your lifestyle choices, and stop killing yourself. If you have been in destructive energy patterns that have been deteriorating your health over time, you can turn things around with your next choice. If there is one thing I have learned after practicing for 20 years and seeing thousands of patients with all types of health problems, it is that as long as you are alive and breathing you have the ability to heal, be healthy, and reach your potential. If you've accumulated damage to different parts of your body, you may need to adjust your human potential pattern and design it to fit within your current capabilities. If running used to feel great and now it causes excruciating pain, switch to power walking, yoga, or riding a bicycle. Work with your health care and crisis care professionals to maximize your mind and body for your next phase of life. Take it on. It's not too late to make the changes you know you need to make. If you need support to make it happen, keep on reading and discover the abundance of resources available to you in the "Health Care Hierarchy" section coming up next.

THE 100-YEAR LIFESTYLE
ACTION PLAN FOR LASTING CHANGE

1. *Stop killing yourself.*
   If you are in a destructive energy pattern, stop now, and stay stopped with every choice from this moment on.

2. *Trust your body.*
   As you begin to turn things around with your choices, your body and mind will strengthen. You will feel yourself getting sharper and younger in mind and body. This will give you the confidence to continue.

3. *Take care of your original parts.*
   Strengthen your weaknesses and adapt your activities to accommodate any areas of your body that are having challenges. Better to change your activities than drive your body parts into submission.

4. *Don't just treat your crisis.*
   Make self-care and health care a priority. Meet with the appropriate health care providers and develop a game plan to maximize your 100-Year Lifestyle while taking into consideration your personal history. Get a second or even a third opinion until the recommendations feel right in your gut, because once again, deep down, you know what is best for you.

5. *Also, learn your family history and become proactive with your health.*
   Make self-care and health care a priority specifically as it relates to your family history.

6. *Remember the three Life-Changing Principles.*
   Change is easy; thinking about change is hard. It is much easier to make the changes for your quality of life, with every choice that supports your ideal 100-Year Lifestyle, than it is to continue on a destructive path and be forced to change by serious disease.

7. *Get excited about what is possible from your current starting point.*
   Look to make progress every day and be careful not to compare yourself to when you were 18 or 35. Get better and feel younger every day through your choices.

PART 4

The Health Care **Hierarchy** of the **100-Year Lifestyle**

When it comes to the old saying "if it ain't broke don't fix it," we need to redefine broke.

CHAPTER 7
CONSUMER-DRIVEN CHANGE IN THE HEALTH CARE INDUSTRY

Consumer demand is powerful and it is rapidly changing our health care industry. Consider the way babies are born today. Many women opt for natural childbirth and have their husbands with them in the delivery rooms. This was not the case a generation or two ago, when the 69 million baby boomers were born. Back then, fathers waited in reception rooms—pacing back and forth, smoking cigarettes, and waiting for the news that baby and mom made it through. Today, smoking is taboo and childbirth is viewed as a much more intimate and natural experience. We are also seeing an increasing number of holistic birthing centers. Midwives and birthing coaches such as doulas—who represent centuries of birthing tradition—are often contracted to provide a natural form of support that is known to shorten labor times. One of the biggest consumer-driven phenomena in recent history is the rise in popularity of organic foods.

GOING ORGANIC
The rise in organic foods is a direct response to consumer demand. This healthy, chemical-free method of growing fruits and vegetables is now a $20-plus billion industry worldwide and it is just beginning to gain momentum. North America has overtaken Europe as the largest market for organic foods. And the term "organic" doesn't apply only to fruits and veggies these days. We are also choosing organic meats, eggs, dairy products, oils, flours, and salad dressings. Organic yogurts and salad bars are making

their way into the public schools, and restaurants featuring organic specialties are sprouting up in cities and towns nationwide. We are even starting to go organic when it comes to our pets. Organic pet foods are growing at nearly three times the rate of conventional foods even though they can be substantially more expensive.

> **Centenarian Secret** There are more than 865 registered pesticides in the United States. Around 350 of those are used on the food we eat. There are 800 products on store shelves across the country—toothpaste, sodas, cookies, vitamins—that contain artificial sweeteners that are suspected of causing many symptoms from dizziness, to seizures, brain tumors, and migraines.

Just a decade ago, eating organic often meant driving miles out of your way to a health food store. And it was hard to even find one. When I opened my first chiropractic office 20 years ago, there was only one within a five-mile radius—and that was in the heart of Atlanta, a big city. At the health food store, choices were limited and, well, not quite as vibrant or appealing as I would have liked. Battered and bruised apples were close to twice the price of conventional ones that were much shinier after being grown and treated with pesticides.

By comparison, organic today has gone from "crunchy" to mainstream. Whole Foods is revolutionizing the grocery business by mainstreaming healthier food solutions. Whole Foods is considered high-end, but nevertheless consumers are flocking to their grocery stores in droves. This consumer demand is driving competitors to begin stocking up on organic as well. Advances in farming and distribution technology are helping to make this possible. As the demand for organic foods continues to increase, the competition and the pricing will make them more affordable for all.

FROM ALTERNATIVE TREATMENTS TO MAINSTREAM HEALTH CARE LEADERS

We are also demanding more holistic care for our minds and bodies. As a result, health care options that are complementary to traditional medical care are rapidly growing. JAMA published a landmark study in 1998, which revealed that four out of ten Americans used alternative health care in the year prior, spending $21.2 billion. The growth of the holistic health care industry has been well documented in Paul Zane Pilzer's books *The Wellness Revolution* and *The Next Trillion*, where he demonstrates how this industry will soon be generating over a trillion dollars in revenue per year.

Slowly but surely, health insurance and managed-care companies are starting to meet the demands of a public that is hungry for these services and willing to pay for them out-of-pocket, when necessary. Expect to see this increase as more and more people realize they are ultimately responsible for their own health. Obviously, this isn't the most desirable outcome, and public pressure is influencing coverage.

Approximately one-third of HMOs now cover chiropractic care. Just under a third cover acupuncture, and a small percentage cover massage therapy. However, most insurance companies do not cover supplementation, exercise equipment, personal training sessions, or nutritional consultations. Still, if these are changes you need to make to ensure your quality of life, you should see them as an investment in your health, assume the responsibility, and incorporate them into your life. After all, not using these types of health care services hurts you and nobody else.

By 2020, expect to see the term *integrative health care* supersede alternative and complementary medicine, with definitive results surrounding certain therapies, leading to their standardization. Expect to see conventional medicine continue its focus on crisis care, with integrative health care focusing on overall health and wellness. Also expect to see society continue to challenge the current system and demand the best from health care providers and technology. This is ultimately good for society and it will be good for you.

Consumers are also taking more control over their standard traditional health care—with good reason. There is simply so much information available today—on the news, in books, and through Web sites like 100yearlifestyle.com, Mercola.com, and WebMD, to name just a few. It's incredible how much information is out there—on everything from the most traditional to the most unconventional ways to take care of yourself. As a result, the paradigm has shifted. People are oftentimes more educated about their options than their doctors. We now want to consult with our doctors and specialists not as gods, but as experts in their field who can give you their opinion. But we want to be the final decision-makers and we've found an unlikely ally to support us in the process: insurance providers. Insurers are starting to arm patients with knowledge, believing that a well-informed patient is a cost-effective patient. One just started offering a wireless information service to policyholders. Patients can look up prices online at the doctor's office via cell phone and debate cost-effective alternatives so they can make informed decisions.

The 100-Year Lifestyle is about so much more, however, than cost-effective, high-tech crisis management.

PUTTING THE "HEALTH" BACK IN HEALTH CARE

Taking control of our own health care—but more importantly, our health—is an important aspect of the 100-Year Lifestyle. After all, why get to 100 if you don't have the mind and body to enjoy it? You'll want to maintain optimum health to enjoy a great quality of life. But you may be asking yourself how you can utilize all of the new information and resources to make the most of it. How does it all fit together?

"Health care" as we know it today, in this country, is largely crisis care. Your physician is largely there to help you detect and solve crises. In this respect, they are kind of like debt counselors. A debt counselor can play a vital role in helping you solve a financial crisis and get you back on track financially. But a debt counselor is not likely able to maximize the growth of your assets, or help you with your IRA, 401(k), or long-term financial planning.

Now, let's say you are in pursuit of financial freedom. How big a role will that debt counselor play toward your ultimate goal? A debt counselor might do a great job getting you on track if you're way off course managing your money. You might pick up the foundation you need, but in order to build up sufficient reserves and become wealthy, you are going to have to master additional knowledge and utilize wealth-building resources. For example, you may need to speak with a financial planner and nurture this relationship as you grow. This type of specialist is not focused on bailing you out, but rather, they work with you on building up your reserves—in this case, cash reserves and assets. This applies to your health as well, building your health reserves every day and avoiding "crisis care" for as long as possible throughout your lifetime.

How do you do this? How do you make sense of all of the information that is out there? How does it all fit together? And most importantly, how can you utilize the information to make the rest of your life the best? That is where the Health Care Hierarchy of the 100-Year Lifestyle comes into play. You'll be able to use this information to set priorities, goals, and take action to support the quality of life you desire and deserve.

THE HEALTH CARE HIERARCHY OF THE 100-YEAR LIFESTYLE

There are three levels to the Health Care Hierarchy of the 100-Year Lifestyle, as follows:

1. *Self-Care:* What you must do for yourself to keep your mind, body, and spirit healthy and functioning at your highest level, which nobody else can do for you.
2. *Health Care:* What you must do for yourself to keep your mind, body, and spirit healthy and functioning at your highest level—utilizing the skills of a trained health care professional.
3. *Crisis Care:* What you must do for yourself to recover from an injury or illness that requires the support of a crisis care or health care specialist.

To achieve a healthy 100-Year Lifestyle, it is important to make self-care and health care your lifestyle, and to prevent the crisis for as long as possible. This actually all goes back to what we discussed earlier—the Titration Principle. When you focus on building health reserves every day—the same as you do financial reserves—the quality of your life will improve every day. Maybe this will require you to defer a little short-term pleasure for long-term benefit. On the upside, it's generally cheaper over time. But it requires you to be motivated by something greater than a crisis.

Identify the things you like doing in the realm of self-care and try to do them every day. I'm going to provide you with a lot of examples in the following chapter. Will they make you feel good and improve your health? Absolutely—they will not only make you feel good today, but also help you stay healthy tomorrow. That's as good as money in the bank and a chronic, healthy smile on your face.

CHAPTER 8
SELF-CARE: MAKING YOUR QUALITY OF LIFE A PRIORITY

Self-care is about taking care of yourself, your mind, body, and spirit. It's about you being responsible for you and doing the things that you know are good for you. Good self-care works with your body's natural ability to be healthy, adapt to stress, maintain strong resistance to disease, and stay in balance. Be good to yourself and make self-care your lifestyle.

This includes eating the foods that you know are right for you, drinking clean water, and breathing clean air. Good self-care includes managing your physique, your energy, and your stress level, and participating in activities that are healthy. Have fun doing things that make you feel strong and vibrant every day.

Many people think that self-care is hard. But this isn't true. Self-care isn't hard—it's actually easy. What *can* be hard is changing your pattern from a destructive or complacent one to a human potential pattern. Remember Change Principle Number 1: Change is easy—thinking about change is hard. Being on the fence is hard. Going back and forth from "should I?" to "shouldn't I?" is hard. The reality is that roller coaster crisis management is the hardest of all.

Undoubtedly, self-care can be time-consuming, but that's where the section on "Quality Time Living" comes in down the road. The truth is, however, you are spending the time anyway— why not spend it with your ideal 100-Year Lifestyle in mind? Great self-care will give you more time by enhancing your energy, strength, and focus. You'll need less sleep and have more energy and personal confidence.

Self-care is about the choices you make every day—thinking healthy thoughts, cultivating high-quality relationships, meditating, and maintaining an exercise routine. If taking care of yourself has not been your norm, its time to start now before a crisis occurs. This may mean making some positive changes that impact your life one choice at a time. One healthy food choice will lead to another. A good workout will inspire you to have another one. Be consistent and eventually you'll feel that you've found your path and your results will motivate you to get to the next level. Do the right things and eventually they will become your new human potential pattern.

Constantly explore new avenues to keep it fun and interesting. If you love yoga, try hot yoga—a style that detoxifies the body. Other popular self-care activities include strength training, sports, gardening, running, aerobics, meditating, attending seminars, listening to music or audio books, taking vacations, swimming, sailing, spiritual retreats, spas, reading, and Pilates, to name a few. You'll know your routine is working for you when it doesn't feel like work. It should be fun and refresh your mind, body, and spirit. You will refine your ideal self-care routine as time goes on.

In addition to keeping your body and mind strong, self-care keeps your immune system strong so your resistance to infections

▶ **LIVE LONG AND STRONG EXERCISE**
The self-care that I want to incorporate into my lifestyle immediately is:

1. _____

2. _____

3. _____

4. _____

5. _____

stays high. Maintaining your resistance is a key component of the 100-Year Lifestyle. Have you ever noticed that healthy people are less likely to get sick than sickly people? Sickly people attract disease. Their bodies become better hosts for diseases to flourish. Keeping yourself healthy with the discipline of great self-care and health care is a much better option. This chapter will cover in detail just some of the practices you can adopt to execute self-care.

EXERCISE: GET YOUR ESS IN SHAPE

Regular exercise is an important part of self-care and nobody can do it for you. It keeps our minds and bodies healthy. If you are not currently exercising, are you waiting to be forced into it by a crisis? If you are already exercising, take it to the next level by getting your ESS in shape. Your ESS is made up of your endurance, strength, and structure. Getting your ESS in shape is important for longevity.

Endurance

Would you trust your body to take you on a long-distance trek in an emergency? If you had to count on your body to save a loved one who needed you to be physically strong, would you be able to? If you had to run away to escape danger, could you? Your endurance is important for all these activities, and it is important for longevity.

If your endurance is high, you will enjoy a great sense of stamina and activity while you age. Your energy will be high and you will feel like doing things. You will not be left home alone while your partner goes off to experience the world. You can increase your stamina through cardiovascular, aerobic exercise that strengthens your heart, burns calories, and increases your energy. Running, cycling, swimming, and power walking are just a few examples of types of exercise that will increase your endurance.

If you already have arthritic or prearthritic conditions, low-impact exercise becomes more and more important as you age. This is why equipment such as elliptical machines, bicycles, rowing machines, and stair-steppers are so popular with people over

50 years of age. They let you exercise your cardiovascular and muscular systems without pounding your joints and your spine.

> **Centenarian Secret**   Set goals for your endurance and continue to challenge yourself. Increase the length of time that you spend doing cardiovascular exercise by 10 percent each month for the next three months and increase your pace as well. If you are not an experienced exerciser, make sure you consult with a certified personal trainer who can customize an endurance plan especially for you.

Cardiovascular exercise is very important to keep your heart and lungs healthy, eliminate stress, and strengthen your immune system. Always exercise with a heart monitor to maximize your results and achieve your goals, while also ensuring that you exercise safely within the normal ranges for your age.

Calculate your target heart rate by age

AGE:	20	30	40	50	60	70
50%	100	95	90	85	80	75
80%	160	152	144	136	128	120

The American Council on Exercise has created this guideline for people up to the age of seventy. With the 100-Year Lifestyle, you and I will create the standard for future generations.

Strength

Strength training is also important for healthy aging because you are going to want and need your muscles to be strong to keep you confident in your body and maintain your independence. If you have good strength, you are more likely to be self-sufficient and independent. Strength training can be done through weights, yoga, Pilates, PowerCentering, and many other styles of exercise. If you set goals for strength training and continually strive to achieve them, you will be excited to see that your strength can increase as you age. Your muscles can stay strong and defined. The sagging skin and muscles we often associate with aging come from not keeping your body toned through strength-training exercise.

If you are already an experienced strength trainer and have a routine already, shake it up a little bit. Try increasing your weight by 10 percent to 20 percent. Get somebody to spot you if necessary and try to squeeze out a few more reps. Vary your exercises on each body part. Work out with a partner and challenge each other. You will begin to see a better result. Always maintain good posture when you strength train to ensure that your spine stays healthy during your training.

We've all heard the expression "if you don't use it, you lose it." This is absolutely true with your strength. Once again, if you have not been actively involved in a strength-training program, consult with a health professional and customize a program.

Structure

Your structure includes your body shape and physical frame. Keeping your structure in shape will keep you looking good and help to prevent injuries while you exercise. Is your waist the size that you desire it to be? How about your arms, your chest, and your legs? Have you measured yourself lately and set goals for your structure so that it is in the shape you desire over your lifetime? You can measure your structure with your eyes at first and decide how you want to change your shape, or get a tape measure and record your measurements. This will give you a starting point for your goals. Measure your neck, biceps, chest, waist, thighs, and calves. If you do not include your structure in your fitness regime, you will find that you start exercising to get in shape, but your shape stays the same as it was before, only you will be a smaller version of yourself. If you are pear shaped and just start doing endurance training, you will become a smaller pear. To truly jump-start you in the direction of your ideal shape, visit a fitness professional and have them develop a program for you.

Another important part of your structure is your spine and posture. A simple way to test its condition is by doing a weight balance test. Rather than stepping on one scale and measuring your weight, you can use two scales and put one foot on each scale. Have somebody else read the numbers for you because if you look down you will tend to sway and throw off your readings. If you are more than three pounds difference on one side of your body compared to the other, you will be putting unnecessary strain on your structure when you exercise.

When I was in full-time practice I used to attend a lot of 5K and 10K road races and volunteer my time to examine the runners. I couldn't believe how many of them were out of balance. It was very common to see people that were ten pounds heavier on one side of their body compared to the other. That's like carrying a bowling ball on one of your hips. Over time this can lead to repetitive strain injuries and serious spinal problems that are

▶ LIVE LONG AND STRONG EXERCISE
100-Year Lifestyle Fitness Assessment: Get Your ESS in Shape

Endurance: Do at least 30 minutes of cardiovascular training three to four times a week. Exercise with a heart monitor and monitor your baseline. Get a personal trainer or other health professional to monitor your progress and get you started on the right track.

Strength: Evaluate the strength of your major muscle groups, including your chest muscles, back muscles, arms, and legs. Set goals for building your strength in each of these areas and get a personal trainer or other health professional to get you started on the right track.

Structure: Measure your neck, chest, waist, hips, and thighs. Evaluate your posture and your weight balance. Set goals for your shape in each of these areas and get a personal trainer, chiropractor, or other health professional to start you on the right track.

Get a 100-Year Lifestyle Fitness Assessment. Measure your current endurance, strength, and structure. Customize an exercise program for yourself and set goals. Keep yourself active, strong, and balanced as you age.

completely preventable if you just keep your structure in balance. I used to love to see people's posture change and their bodies get back into balance within a few adjustments and have them rave about the improvements to their running. Many professional athletes incorporate adjustments into their regular training routine for this reason, as well as to improve recovery time between games and practices, and to speed the healing time of injuries. Balance is crucial to being able to enjoy exercise for the long haul. Weight balance is an important part of healthy exercise and properly caring for your physical structure.

If you really want to get your ESS in shape, make the commitment to see your fitness professional today and ask for your 100-Year Lifestyle Fitness Assessment, which can be downloaded from 100yearlifestyle.com.

Also, pay attention to your chairs, mattresses, and bedding, particularly as you age. You want them to support your spine. They should support the natural curvature of your neck and back. You will start to feel like you are old when you start to feel old physically because your body gets stiff, sore, and tight. It's hard to believe, but we actually spend a third of our lives lying down—sleeping. If you sleep eight hours a night and you live to 100, you will spend 33 years in a bed. And if you are like many of us and have a desk job, you probably spend close to another third sitting. This is why ergonomic chairs that support your body properly are an important component of self-care.

A good bed will not be too hard, and it won't be too soft either. Like the porridge in the "Goldilocks and the Three Bears" nursery rhyme, it will be just right. Many bed manufacturers today have technology that can measure the pressure in your spine when you lay down on a bed to see how it fits your body. Using a pillow that supports the natural curve in your neck is also important to ensure its stability and to keep pressure off of your nerves. Your chiropractor can take a simple X-ray of your neck to show you how your neck is positioned so that you can make the appropriate choices for your long-term well-being. You should be able to personalize your side of the bed so that you and your spouse can both enjoy the refreshing feeling of a good night's sleep, consistently.

Ergonomically designed chairs, computer workstations, and work platforms are important to ensure that you don't injure yourself on the job. When I got into practice in the mid-eighties, the science of ergonomics was barely known in the work world. Today, it is hard to find a responsible company that does not take ergonomics into consideration for their employees. Be responsible for your own safety, however, with good self-care on the job. If you sit at a computer for any length of time, make sure that your knees are at a 90-degree bend and your feet are flat on the floor or slightly elevated. Make sure your spine is straight and your shoulders hang comfortably, keeping your lower arms parallel to the floor.

Always lift with your legs and not your back. Statistics show that 80 percent of the population will have a severe episode of back pain at some point in their life. Good self-care and health care choices will keep you healthy and prevent you from feeling old before your time.

PROVIDE YOUR BODY WITH EXTRA PROTECTION FROM HARMFUL SUBSTANCES

The air in your environment will be inside your body when you breathe. The water in your home and the places where you dine will also be ingested and become a part of your body. If you want to help your body stay healthy, keep them clean.

Use Air and Water Filters

Just recently my son had some friends over to the house for a party and since it was winter, I thought it would be nice to light up the fireplace. Little did I know that some creature had built a nest in our chimney, and before we knew it the entire house was filled up with smoke. We had to evacuate the house, open all the windows and doors, and let the house air out.

When all the visible smoke had cleared, we went back inside and, unfortunately, the smell was very present and we could feel the ill effects by the next morning. I went out and bought two air filters and ran them in the house the next few days, and I was thrilled at how well they worked. I stopped taking the air that we breathe for granted after that episode.

Air pollution is a problem in the United States, so use air filters, wash your bedding often, and follow smog alerts. Avoid exercising outside on smoggy days, and consider cutting back on all the lawn chemical treatments. In many parts of the country, having a lawn that looks "golf-course good" is the new standard. Unfortunately, many of those chemicals are highly toxic. Consider organic alternatives. Airborne toxins affect our health in a variety of ways and come in a variety of forms:

Ozone:
The major component of smog and most pervasive air pollutants, this poisonous allotrope can cause severe coughing, shortness of breath, pained breathing, lung and eye irritation, and greater susceptibility to pneumonia, bronchitis, and other respiratory illnesses.

Dioxin:
One of the most potent animal carcinogens ever tested, dioxin can cause severe weight loss, liver problems, kidney problems, birth defects, and death.

Nitrogen Oxide:
A major component of acid rain. It can damage lung tissue.

Volatile Organic Compounds:
These compounds are generated by power plants, motor vehicles, and waste combustors. They are associated with cancer, and neurological and reproductive problems.

Natural Allergens:
Allergens (like pollen and fungal spores) can contribute to increased rates of asthma, allergies, and respiratory conditions when your body is not functioning properly.

Drink Purified Water

One of the very best things you can do for your health is to drink purified water. This means investing in water filters for your home and investing in highly purified bottled water. Sure, a gallon of clean water can be even more expensive than a gallon of gasoline, which is a shame—but it's worth it.

> **Centenarian Secret** According to UNICEF, A child dies every 15 seconds from disease attributable to unsafe drinking water, deplorable sanitation, and poor hygiene.

In the United States, pesticides, fertilizers, animal excrement, bacteria, oil spills, radiation, and other toxins also make their way into our ground water supply. In fact, about one-third of the U.S. drinking water supply tested recently by the Natural Resources Defense Council showed the presence of arsenic, bacteria, organic chemicals, and other substances. Cumulative exposure can cause cancer as well as vomiting, abdominal pain, and other problems. The quick and easy disposal of waste in this country—again, another short-term gain—threatens our collective long-term health.

Avoid Toxic Chemicals

Your body is a collection of chemicals—from the hydrochloric acid that breaks down the food in your stomach to the oxygen that converts it into energy and the minerals that nourish your organs. When these processes are balanced and regulated properly by your nervous, immune, and hormonal systems, your body has the ability to minimize the effects of these toxins and fight off disease. Unfortunately, the acid, pH, iron, and other chemical levels in your body can become out of balance, negatively affecting your health. External irritants can overwhelm your body's natural coping mechanisms, especially if your body is out of balance to begin with. Many of the irritants and toxins are invisible, and we really don't choose to have them enter our bodies. Keeping your body strong and healthy with great self-care and health care will keep your body in the best condition possible to resist their negative impact and cleanse them from your system.

Centenarian Secret   According to the <u>Journal of American Medicine</u>, tobacco use killed more people in the United States in 2000 than any other substance. Approximately 435,000 people died from the cumulative effects of tobacco exposure, 85,000 died from alcohol-related illnesses, and another 17,000 from using illegal drugs.

Tobacco, alcohol, and illegal drugs all cause chemical toxicity that can interfere with the body's natural ability to be healthy. But so do many over-the-counter and prescription drugs. Every year, more than 2 million people experience adverse drug reactions from properly prescribed medications. Nearly 100,000 die from chemical reactions to ordinary medicines you might find in your own bathroom cabinet. One of the reasons why this is so prevalent today is that we believe a magic pill exists for all of our ills. Too often, we reach for medications to dull our pain, alter our children's behavior, increase our libido, or enhance our athletic prowess without a second thought as to their side effects. The problem is that we are often risking our long-term health for a short-term gain.

Over-the-counter and prescription drugs can cause adverse side effects like organ deterioration, organ dysfunction, and possible death. Many people have the notion that over-the-counter medications must be completely safe, but in reality, we all need to use caution when taking any type of medicine. Take it only when necessary and when other holistic solutions have been ineffective. Beware of their side effects, study the contraindications, and don't exceed the recommended dosage. Consider holistic self-care and health care options whenever possible and use medications as a last resort.

According to the Centers for Education and Research on Therapeutics, over 2 million people experience serious adverse drug reactions each year. Also, according to the National Center for Immunization and Respiratory Diseases, tens of millions of antibiotic prescriptions are written for viral infections that they are unable to treat.

Continuous exposure to any type of toxin will force your body into a chronic stress reaction—draining your energy over time and distracting your body from its genetic goals. As it moves into and stays in a reactive mode in an attempt to ward off the side effects of these toxins, your body can move into survival and shut down. Why not prevent this and keep yourself pure with good filtration.

MANAGE STRESS

Managing stress is a key component of the 100-Year Lifestyle. A benefit of our extended life span is the knowledge that we can survive the challenges that life throws our way.

Your body is adaptable, with remarkable capacities to heal. Empower it as much as you can through your lifestyle. Nurture and cultivate your health reserves, much like your savings account. This way, you'll be prepared to handle everything the future brings—which you can count on as being a mixture of good and bad—joyous times and challenging ones. Knowing that you have survived thus far will keep you from suffering extreme ups and downs that can increase your stress unnecessarily. Decide whether you will be the kind of person that makes a situation better or worse when you are exposed to a challenge. Having faith that you will make the most of every situation will certainly bring you through the challenging times and help you come out on top.

Think about all the events or issues that we have worried about over the first half, or first two-thirds of our life. Isn't it great to know that we have come through them all with the wisdom and confidence that we will survive and maybe even come out better from the experience? Combining this wisdom and maturity with the fully developed talents and the inner knowledge about ourselves is another aspect of the 100-Year Lifestyle that is exciting and can help us to manage stress more effectively, and the benefits are many. I'll discuss methods that can be used to achieve these benefits in the following sections.

Meditation

You can achieve a reduced stress level through practices like meditation. Meditation focuses your thoughts and produces a sense of calm. Over time, meditation can strengthen coping mechanisms in a crisis. Meditation requires regular practice—generally, once or twice a day for 20 to 30 minutes is sufficient. When you meditate, you are fully alert but you are not focused on the outside world. Instead, you cultivate inner awareness. You get to this state by focusing your mind on one thing—your breath, a single word, or an inspirational passage. Meditation is focused concentration and can even be done while exercising.

The best time to meditate is when you are free from distraction. This means when you are feeling fresh, comfortable, and relaxed. It can be a great way to start, break up, or end your day. It is often recommended that you stretch before you meditate, then take a seated position and assume a chosen meditation posture. This may be cross-legged on the floor, or sitting up straight in a chair. You can also meditate lying flat on your back with your palms facing up. Close your eyes. Start to breathe in and breathe out—slowly and deeply. Count to seven or eight on each inhale and then again on each exhale. Make sure that you have good posture if you are sitting. Focusing on your breath is generally sufficient for producing a meditative state.

If you are just getting started, you may consider buying some guided meditation tapes. There are many excellent books and tapes to choose from that will help you get started.

Try Yoga

The best way to get acquainted with yoga is by trying out some classes and picking up an issue of one of the many excellent yoga magazines on bookshelves everywhere. There are myriad videotapes and DVDs available. However, you need to get a sense of the industry to find the levels, practices, and instructors that work for you. At its best, yoga quiets the mind, improves your concentration, stretches the muscles, and even massages internal organs. When you leave a good yoga class, you are glowing.

A good yoga instructor will gently guide you toward achieving optimal postures. A great yoga instructor will also focus on creating an optimal setting for your instruction. They know that you should feel relaxed and safe. Many instructors will dim the lights and use candles. They will carefully choose their music before each class. Their voices should be calming and nurturing. Yoga, along with all of the self-care and health care strategies discussed here, can make you feel younger and healthier within just a few weeks.

> **Centenarian Secret** Excessive stress shortens our lives, leads to chronic health problems, and also negatively impacts our relationships, work, and quality of life. Should you have something routinely stressing you right now, practice stress management—this will help you get centered and find optimal ways to handle it.

Retreats

Self-care is about nurturing and nourishing your mind, body, and spirit. There are countless ways to do this. The important thing is that you choose activities that you enjoy doing and that you do them regularly.

You might consider exploring new ideas at a spa. High-quality spas are all about great self-care and they will expose you to so many options to choose from. You'll learn meditation, chi gong, tai chi, power walking meditation, and yoga. For a super dose of self-care, spas are a superb solution. They remove you from your daily stresses and catapult you into the ultimate self-care experience. If you have never been to a spa that is completely dedicated to your self-care—with on-site health care providers whose purpose is to remove every ounce of stress from your body—you are really missing out. Everyone should go to a spa for at least one three-day weekend a year to break away and rejuvenate the spirit. If your finances permit (see Financing Your 100-Year Lifestyle later in the book), visit a spa at least once a quarter. The top spas around the world not only rejuvenate your mind, body, and spirit, but they also educate you on how to bring the 100-Year Lifestyle principles home with you.

As I travel around the world teaching these concepts to companies, health conscious individuals, and health care providers, I have noticed over the past few years how hotel chains have incorporated self-care amenities into their basic packages. In an effort to improve customer loyalty, the Starwood Hotel chain has upgraded to the Heavenly Bed and Westin Workouts powered by Reebok. Marriott just introduced Revive, their bed and relaxation system, and Hyatt and all of the other quality hotel chains are also upgrading their self-care systems to keep up and maintain their share of the market. They realize that the best way for them to care for their customers is to provide them with all of the self-care resources while they are on the road away from home. While spas used to be, and still can be, exclusive for the rich and famous, spa facilities are available at nearly all hotel chains. They need to provide these types of services in order to compete.

KEEP AN EYE ON YOUR SELF-CARE

How do you know if you are letting your self-care slip? You are probably overweight, overstressed, and are not getting enough rest. You are probably eating too much fast food and not taking enough time to slow down and balance your life. You are motivated by crisis and you only take care of yourself when you feel pain or you get sick. You find yourself on a crisis roller coaster, living from one challenge to the next, defining your life by these crises. You may even find yourself telling these crisis stories over and over and over again to your family and friends. Maybe you are taking constant trips to the drugstore, trying to mask symptoms rather than making trips to the gym, taking walks, visiting your local health food store, or visiting your health care providers for regular wellness visits.

Creating your own personal human potential pattern for your self-care and health care will help you ensure the highest quality of life you desire.

CHAPTER 9
HEALTH CARE: BUILDING A QUALITY OF LIFE HEALTH CARE TEAM

ealth care is a proactive way to keep your body and mind as healthy as possible. Health care is the care you cannot provide for yourself. It is necessary to keep your body balanced, aligned, stress free, and better able to resist the challenges of your environment. Just like you cannot do surgery on yourself in times of a crisis, there are many aspects of health care that are necessary to keep you functioning at your highest level that you can not do for yourself. For example, you cannot massage yourself, but massage is important to keep your muscles and your lymphatic system healthy and to eliminate the accumulation of stress from your body. You cannot adjust your own spine, but wellness chiropractic care is important to keep your spine and nervous system healthy throughout your lifetime. There are also times when you have difficulty thinking clearly about things—when it would be helpful to talk with a life coach, therapist, or a counselor. Maybe you've leveled off on the results you are getting from your exercise program, so you decide to consult with a personal trainer. Or it could be that you are having a difficult time with your diet and you would benefit from consulting a nutritionist. Building a health care team to keep you in the best shape of your life is the true purpose of health care according to the 100-Year Lifestyle.

TAKE CARE OF YOUR MIND AND BODY
In my practice, I found that people who are committed to a human potential pattern of self-care and health care almost always respond

better to a crisis. For example, I worked with a family that had a couple of severe health issues. The mother had reoccurring headaches and one of her children had juvenile rheumatoid arthritis. Within a month of beginning their chiropractic care, both the mom and daughter felt much better and through the educational program we provided, they began making healthier choices overall. They continued with their care to achieve optimum function of their spine and nervous system even after they felt better and made this a part of their health care. They started on a wellness adjustment plan as well as an overall wellness plan focusing on good nutrition and exercise. Over time, their bodies began to heal and function much better on every level. The mother told me that she felt better than she had in years. Her daughter no longer needed the drugs that were beginning to cause very annoying and unhealthy side effects. She was back on the swim team and they were ecstatic about her health.

Her husband, however, did not share in her joy. While he was glad that everyone was feeling better, he was not supportive of the new health care routines. He was strictly motivated by crisis and did not see the value of self-care and ongoing health care. Well, unfortunately, one day the family was involved in a car accident. The entire family was in the car and experienced the same impact. They were all injured in similar ways, feeling the effects of the whiplash, but it was the husband who took the longest to recover. The rest of the family healed readily and suffered less. The benefits of his family's self-care and health care became evident to him as a result of this crisis. He became a convert, moving from a crisis-motivated junkie to a self-care, health care, quality-of-life motivated man. What a difference it made in his life, and what a difference it will make in yours.

Health care is about health and wellness, and keeping your body strong. First of all, you need to understand that your body is designed to be healthy. Disease is not a normal part of everyday life. When it happens, it is unfortunate, but we need to stop thinking of sickness as natural. This is like assuming that debt and bankruptcy are normal. They are not. Now, they can happen.

And if they do, it's nice to know there is a system in place to get us back on track. But having to treat a disease is something we would all like to avoid if we can, and in many cases we can.

Excellent health care, combined with great self-care, keeps your entire body functioning at its optimum level. While we all brush our teeth and floss after each meal (don't we?), we still see our dentist at least once or twice a year for a thorough examination. Dentistry was the first profession that packaged self-care, health care, and crisis care so that it made sense to the consumer. Most people clearly understand the value of keeping your teeth healthy, clean, and white while avoiding the dreaded root canal.

Centenarian Secret The Top 5 Traits of Successful Exercisers by Mike Epstein, CPT, VP of Gold's Gym, Paramus, New Jersey, Board of Director, Gold's Gym International:

1. Successful exercisers are motivated.
2. Successful exercisers educate themselves and seek professional assistance.
3. Successful exercisers set small, obtainable, and realistic goals.
4. Successful exercisers make fitness a part of their lifestyle.
5. Successful exercisers use visual feedback to measure their progress.

Chiropractors have also done a terrific job packaging the Health Care Hierarchy for the spine and nervous system. Just like nobody wants a root canal, people would prefer to keep their spine and nervous system healthy, balanced, and aligned throughout their lifetime. They want to be able to stay active as they age. We've all seen an elderly person whose spine is bent over and crooked from years of neglect and said to ourselves, "I don't want to end up like that." These crippled people didn't just wake up like that one day. Their spine grew wrong over time as their nerves deteriorated over time. Haven't you also seen the unfortunate soul who neglected his or her spine and ended up with a herniated or ruptured disk? Ouch. It only takes one bad disk to put a damper on your quality of life as you age. Given the relationship between the spine and nervous system and all of the ill effects that come with preventable spinal problems, no wonder millions of people swear by their chiropractic care and have made it such an important part of their 100-Year Lifestyle. In fact, one of our favorite almost centenarians, fitness guru Jack LaLanne, was also trained as a chiropractor.

THE IMPORTANCE OF EARLY DETECTION

Our current medical system is almost all about crisis care. The emphasis on early detection, however, is an important aspect of health care because research has shown that if you are inflicted with a serious illness, early detection increases your chances of recovery. However, early detection won't get you in the best shape of your life and help you avoid the crisis. If it's been detected, you are in crisis. The following pages show a schedule of early detection testing that has been provided by the U.S. Department of Health and Human Services. Since the list can be overwhelming and many of these tests are unnecessary for everyone, follow the recommendations, making those areas that you know are a part of your family history a priority. For example, if heart disease runs in your family, make early detection examinations with a cardiologist. Your physician will monitor your cholesterol levels and blood pressure to help you avoid heart disease. If they are high, your doctor will talk to you about changes you need to make to your diet. This may mean fewer eggs, leaner meats, more fruits and vegetables, and less sodium. However, if you find that these recommendations are limited, consult a nutritionist. Physicians study little about nutrition in medical school and are more inclined to recommend drugs. Do your homework and look to change your life.

If colon cancer is a part of your history, follow the recommended schedule for screenings and at the same time, eat healthy and take the self-care steps to keep your colon healthy.

Early detection screenings for both men and women include hearing and vision tests, blood pressure checks, cholesterol tests, cancer screening, dental exams, and chiropractic spinal screenings. Men are advised to have an annual prostate check—including a digital rectal examination or a blood test.

Women should have annual breast exams, PAP tests, pelvic exams, and also mammograms. The advice on when some of these tests should be started, and the frequency with which they are given, varies. Work with a trusted health care provider to come up with a plan that works for you. If you get a positive test, you might want to redo the test a second time before you panic. False positives are not uncommon. Also, always consider getting second opinions on any course of action, as you would be amazed how opinions can vary from one provider to the next. We found this to be true firsthand when my wife, Lisa, was pregnant with our oldest son, Jacob. Her blood sugar was slightly elevated and our initial obstetrician recommended radical and aggressive procedures to monitor her blood sugar. We did not agree with his recommendations. Our personal research and gut feeling told us that this was unnecessary, and we went on a search for a second and third opinion. We found that the differences between obstetricians were massive. Finally we came upon a doctor who we felt was right on in his recommendations. We monitored her blood sugar through nutrition and exercise, and Jacob was born a healthy baby. We avoided an intensely aggressive protocol with a much higher risk of side effects.

Just as important, if not more important, is exercising your heart, eating healthy, and making your self-care a priority.

PREVENTION

Many people confuse early detection with prevention. There is a big difference. Early detection consists of engaging in diagnostic testing for the purpose of identifying a condition in its earliest stages. This is not the same as prevention, which is what a healthy 100-Year Lifestyle can help you achieve. Millions of people have a chiropractor or nutritionist as their primary health care specialist and a physician as their crisis care specialist.

One interesting side note is important as I write this section. I can hear the voices on the extremes of the antimedical side

screaming about all of the medical mishaps that happen and saying that they would never go to a medical doctor or have any of
these tests. Interestingly, I have seen dozens of these people end
up in the hospital and under the knife, having their lives saved by
a dedicated medical professional. Afterward, they often ease their
position as they see how their role is important in the Health
Care Hierarchy.

I have also heard the voices of old-time medical physicians who
for decades badmouthed the chiropractic profession and other up-
and-coming health care providers, such as acupuncturists, massage therapists, personal trainers, nutritionists, and others. Now,
many of them are utilizing their services regularly to stay healthy.
In my practice I saw dozens of physicians and their families who
were committed to regular wellness adjustment plans, and I know
many of my colleagues who do the same. There is an important
place for everyone and at some time or another we may want and
need all of these professionals in our lives.

Health Screening Schedule for Women
From the U.S. Department of Health and
Human Services Office on Women's Health

SCREENING TESTS	AGES 18–39	AGES 40–49	AGES 50–64	AGES 65 AND OLDER
General health: Full checkup, including weight and height	Discuss with your doctor or nurse	Discuss with your doctor or nurse	Discuss with your doctor or nurse	Discuss with your doctor or nurse
Thyroid test (TSH)	Start at age 35, then every 5 years	Every 5 years	Every 5 years	Every 5 years
Heart health: Blood pressure test	At least every 2 years	At least every 2 years	At least every 2 years	At least every 2 years

continued

SCREENING TESTS	AGES 18–39	AGES 40–49	AGES 50–64	AGES 65 AND OLDER
Cholesterol test	Start at age 20; discuss with your doctor or nurse	Discuss with your doctor or nurse	Discuss with your doctor or nurse	Discuss with your doctor or nurse
Bone health: Bone mineral density test	—	Discuss with your doctor or nurse	Discuss with your doctor or nurse	Get a bone mineral density test at least once; Talk to your doctor or nurse about repeat testing
Diabetes: Blood sugar test	Discuss with your doctor or nurse	Start at age 45, then every 3 years	Every 3 years	Every 3 years
Breast health: Mammogram (X-ray of breast)	—	Every 1–2 years; Discuss with your doctor or nurse	Every 1–2 years; Discuss with your doctor or nurse	Every 1–2 years; Discuss with your doctor or nurse
Reproductive health: Pap test and pelvic exam	Every 1–3 years if you have been sexually active or are older than 21	Every 1–3 years	Every 1–3 years	Discuss with your doctor or nurse
Chlamydia test	If sexually active, yearly until age 25; ages 26–39, if you are at high risk for chlamydia or other STDs, you may need this test	If you are at high risk for chlamydia or other STDs, you may need this test	If you are at high risk for chlamydia or other STDs, you may need this test	If you are at high risk for chlamydia or other STDs, you may need this test

continued

SCREENING TESTS	AGES 18–39	AGES 40–49	AGES 50–64	AGES 65 AND OLDER
Sexually transmitted disease (STD) test	Both partners should get tested for STDs, including HIV, before initiating sexual intercourse	Both partners should get tested for STDs, including HIV, before initiating sexual intercourse	Both partners should get tested for STDs, including HIV, before initiating sexual intercourse	Both partners should get tested for STDs, including HIV, before initiating sexual intercourse
Colorectal health: Fecal occult blood test	—	—	Yearly	Yearly
Flexible sigmoidoscopy (with fecal occult blood test is preferred)	—	—	Every 5 years (if not having a colonoscopy)	Every 5 years (if not having a colonoscopy)
Double Contrast Barium Enema	—	—	Every 5–10 years (if not having a colonoscopy or sigmoidoscopy)	Every 5–10 years (if not having a colonoscopy or sigmoidoscopy)
Colonoscopy	—	—	Every 10 years	Every 10 years
Rectal exam	Discuss with your doctor or nurse	Discuss with your doctor or nurse	Every 5–10 years with each screening (sigmoidoscopy, colonoscopy, or DCBE)	Every 5–10 years with each screening (sigmoidoscopy, colonoscopy, or DCBE)

continued

SCREENING TESTS	AGES 18–39	AGES 40–49	AGES 50–64	AGES 65 AND OLDER
Eye and ear health: Eye exam	Get your eyes checked if you have problems or visual changes	Every 2–4 years	Every 2–4 years	Every 1–2 years
Hearing test	Starting at age 18, then every 10 years	Every 10 years	Discuss with your doctor or nurse	Discuss with your doctor or nurse
Skin health: Mole exam	Monthly mole self-exam; by a doctor every 3 years, starting at age 20	Monthly mole self-exam; by a doctor every year	Monthly mole self-exam; by a doctor every year	Monthly mole self-exam; by a doctor every year
Oral health: Dental exam	1–2 times every year	1–2 times every year	1–2 times every year	1–2 times every year
Mental health screening	Discuss with your doctor or nurse	Discuss with your doctor or nurse	Discuss with your doctor or nurse	Discuss with your doctor or nurse

Health Screening Schedule for Men
From the U.S. Department of Health and Human Services

SCREENING TESTS	AGES 18–39	AGES 40–49	AGES 50–64	AGES 65 AND OLDER
General health: Full checkup, including weight and height	Discuss with your doctor or nurse	Discuss with your doctor or nurse	Discuss with your doctor or nurse	Discuss with your doctor or nurse
Heart health: Blood pressure test	At least every 2 years	At least every 2 years	At least every 2 years	At least every 2 years

continued

SCREENING TESTS	AGES 18–39	AGES 40–49	AGES 50–64	AGES 65 AND OLDER
Cholesterol test	Start at age 20; discuss with your doctor or nurse	Discuss with your doctor or nurse	Discuss with your doctor or nurse	Discuss with your doctor or nurse
Diabetes: Blood sugar test	Discuss with your doctor or nurse	Start at age 45, then every 3 years	Every 3 years	Every 3 years
Prostate health: Digital rectal exam (DRE)	—	Discuss with your doctor or nurse	Discuss with your doctor or nurse	Discuss with your doctor or nurse
Prostate-specific antigen (PSA) (blood test)	—	Discuss with your doctor or nurse	Discuss with your doctor or nurse	Discuss with your doctor or nurse
Reproductive health: Testicular exam	Monthly self-exam; and part of a general checkup	Monthly self-exam; and part of a general checkup	Monthly self-exam; and part of a general checkup	Month self-exam; and part of a general checkup
Chlamydia test	Discuss with your doctor or nurse	Discuss with your doctor or nurse	Discuss with your doctor or nurse	Discuss with your doctor or nurse
Sexually transmitted disease (STD) test	Both partners should get tested for STDs, including HIV, before initiating sexual intercourse	Both partners should get tested for STDs, including HIV, before initiating sexual intercourse	Both partners should get tested for STDs, including HIV, before initiating sexual intercourse	Both partners should get tested for STDs, including HIV, before initiating sexual intercourse
Colorectal health	—	—	Yearly	Yearly

continued

SCREENING TESTS	AGES 18–39	AGES 40–49	AGES 50–64	AGES 65 AND OLDER
Flexible sigmoidos-copy (with fecal occult blood test is preferred)	—	—	Every 5 years (if not having a colonoscopy)	Every 5 years (if not having a colonoscopy)
Double con-trast barium enema	—	—	Every 5–10 years (if not having a colonoscopy or sigmoidos-copy)	Every 5–10 years (if not having a colonoscopy or sigmoidos-copy)
Colonoscopy	—	—	Every 10 years	Every 10 years
Rectal exam	Discuss with your doctor or nurse	Discuss with your doctor or nurse	Every 5–10 years with each screen-ing (sig-moidoscopy, colonoscopy, or DCBE)	Every 5–10 years with each screen-ing (sig-moidoscopy, colonoscopy, or DCBE)
Eye and ear health: Eye exam	Get your eyes checked if you have problems or visual changes	Every 2–4 years	Every 2–4 years	Every 1–2 years
Hearing Test	Starting at age 18, then every 10 years	Every 10 years	Discuss with your doctor or nurse	Discuss with your doctor or nurse

continued

SCREENING TESTS	AGES 18–39	AGES 40–49	AGES 50–64	AGES 65 AND OLDER
Skin health: Mole exam	Monthly mole self-exam; by a doctor every 3 years, starting at age 20	Monthly mole self-exam; by a doctor every year	Monthly mole self-exam; by a doctor every year	Monthly mole self-exam; by a doctor every year
Oral health: Dental exam	One to two times every year	One to two times every year	One to two times every year	One to two times every year
Mental health screening	Discuss with your doctor or nurse	Discuss with your doctor or nurse	Discuss with your doctor or nurse	Discuss with your doctor or nurse

PRIMARY HEALTH CARE PROVIDERS

There are many other primary health care providers that you should see who complement the early detection screening work done by your physician. Rather than helping you achieve early detection, they are important for your health and well-being. This includes your nutritionist to keep your diet healthy, your personal trainer to personalize your fitness program, your chiropractor to keep your spine and nervous system healthy, and your dentist to keep your teeth clean. True health care providers work with you on building your reserves and keeping you at the top of your game. They promote your optimum health and wellness.

Dentists, for example, not only help keep your teeth and gums healthy, but they also keep the rest of your body healthy as well. Studies have revealed that good oral health is a factor in maintaining your overall physical well-being. Optometrists help to maintain eye health. They diagnose eye problems and vision disease, prescribe eyeglasses, and can even help you strengthen your eyes with exercises.

Podiatrists provide foot care that is important to your feet, which can affect the structure of your entire body. Orthotics and foot supports, especially ones that are custom designed to your feet, are something that all active people should consider and can be obtained at a variety of places including podiatric offices, shoe stores that sell custom-made shoes, and chiropractic offices, since foot alignment can also effect spinal alignment.

Chiropractic Care

Chiropractic care is a vital health care option that has been misunderstood for its 110-plus year history. It was founded on the principles that are readily accepted by all health care providers today, that human beings have within them an innate intelligence that is self-healing and self-regulating. The body has the ability to stay healthy as long as there is no interference. Initially chiropractors attracted patients who were the sickest of the sick and many of these patients healed miraculously.

While many conditions are helped through chiropractic care, the purpose of the care is to align the spine and remove pressure from the nerve system so the body can heal itself and restore itself to normal function. Research has shown conclusively that when pressure is placed on spinal nerves the body breaks down and when the pressure is removed the body begins to heal. This is why healthy people as well as sick people are attracted to chiropractic care—both as an important part of their crisis care management as well as their health care routine. It is not designed to replace traditional care, but it is designed to be a drug-free, holistic solution on its own—as well as a complement to traditional crisis care.

Many professional athletes and sports teams utilize chiropractic care to recover quickly from injuries and maximize their athletic performance. You hear people all the time say about chiropractic care, "I don't know how people live without it!" Occasionally you will hear the crisis care skeptic say that once you begin chiropractic care you will have to go for the rest of your life. This is not true. There is no "have to." It is just like going to the dentist. If you want to keep your teeth healthy for life, your self-care regimen is to brush and floss your teeth every day and visit your dentist for regular checkups. The better you are at your self-care and health care, the healthier your teeth will be.

Think of chiropractic care this way: you will probably visit a dentist your entire lifetime. The same is true for your chiropractic care. The frequency and intensity of the care you'll require will depend on the amount of self-care you give your spine on a daily basis. Good self-care habits including having good posture, practicing yoga, and doing stretches, as well as good sleeping, sitting, and stress management habits, will ensure that you require less frequent visits to your chiropractor. The more you neglect your self-care, the more frequently you will need to be adjusted. Your frequency of need will also be determined by your history of trauma involving the spine.

Fortunately, chiropractic has grown up over the past 110 years and there are now many types of chiropractic procedures and techniques—from the traditional adjustment where you hear the "sound" of the spine being adjusted to very light touch, soft-tissue techniques by hand or through the use of computer technology and instruments that balance the spine. Some techniques work better for some people than others, but the important thing is to find the one that works best for you and to utilize that care as a part of your overall health care strategy for a lifetime. The best news of all is that chiropractic is one of the safest forms of health care, with extremely low incidences of malpractice and patient injury. Aside from the occasional scare campaign by dinosaur groups, chiropractors work very well with all types of physicians to do what is in the best interest of their patients.

PERSONAL TRAINERS

The personal-training industry has become a field of specialists. If you are an athlete who is striving for peak performance, there are trainers who specialize in that. If you are looking to decrease your body fat to the normal range—12 to 15 percent for men, and 15 to 20 percent for women—there are trainers who can help you with that. If you want to improve your cardiovascular fitness, you can also find trainers who specialize in that. The key to having success with your personal trainer is to clearly communicate your goals.

When you choose a personal trainer, make sure you find one that is certified. There are several professional associations that certify personal trainers and ensure that they are trained properly. Review your exercise program with your trainer every three to six months. Revisit your goals regularly as well, and maintain great communication with your trainer.

> **Centenarian Secret**   There are so many self-care options out there today. New products are being made available and new services are being offered all the time. How do you discern the good from the bad? Industry associations are a good place to start. For example, in the chiropractic profession, we have the International Chiropractors Association, the World Chiropractic Alliance, the American Chiropractic Association, and the Federation of Straight Chiropractors and Organizations. Each organization has a membership base that is in alignment with their philosophy. You can go to their Web sites to learn more about each group and then find referrals.

MASSAGE THERAPISTS

Massage has also been proven to relieve a variety of conditions such as many of the discomforts of pregnancy, like backaches, leg cramps, morning sickness, varicose veins, and headaches. Massage may even be used during labor to ease the pain and potentially shorten the labor. Some studies suggest that massage may also be an effective way to treat PMS. Massage is quickly becoming an accepted way to treat pain. Americans now rate massage equal to pain relievers for efficacy of pain treatment. One in five Americans took advantage of this therapy last year. However, crisis care is only one way to utilize massage. Getting regular massage keeps your body stress free, relaxes you, and can keep you as healthy as possible. Determine the frequency that works best for you and make massage a part of your lifestyle.

NUTRITIONISTS AND DIETICIANS

Good nutrition is another key to good health care. "You are what you eat" is a true statement, since your breakfast in the morning will become a part of your body by the afternoon. Keep yourself healthy with good nutrition. A certified dietician or nutritionist can help you develop an eating plan that fits your lifestyle and your current health condition. They can also help you choose a supplement program that can fill in the gaps of your diet and give you extra support to counterbalance your family history.

Supplementation is important in today's world since most of us don't always eat properly and can be challenged by stress. A good supplement is absorbed into the body so that it can be used by your cells. Blood testing and new technologies that evaluate the health of your cells can determine the effectiveness of your supplementation.

CHAPTER 10
CRISIS CARE: PREPARING FOR AND AVOIDING A CRISIS-FILLED LIFE

At some time or another we will all have a crisis. Being prepared will ensure that our bodies recover as quickly as possible and our pocketbooks recover quickly as well. Having a crisis care team of health care specialists with a primary doctor you can trust is certainly an important part of the process. You will develop this health care team as you explore and practice the self-care and health care elements of the Health Care Hierarchy.

Who is going to pay for your crisis, and for your health care for that matter? Health insurance as we know it today is really crisis protection. If you get sick or injured, your health insurance policy is designed to take care of you. When I first got into practice, it was common for people to have $100 deductible policies with 90 percent coverage. This sure seems like an eternity ago. Contracts now limit coverage, cap costs, and incite managed-care doctors to not recommend certain treatments. On the other hand, we are starting to see coverage for health care options like massage, acupuncture, and chiropractic care to help you in times of crisis.

Insurance companies are trying to adapt to a changing marketplace, but if you or a loved one has had a health crisis in the past decade or so, you are likely to have had some issues with your insurer. And all of us have experienced rising costs and declining benefits. How many times have you changed insurance companies over the past 20 or so years? How many times have your policy premiums changed? Have your premiums gone up? Mine sure have. Have your benefits gone down? You're not alone—we are all in the same boat.

The take-away from all of this is not to try to make sense of a system that isn't always working. This is tricky, as we have a paternalistic view of the health care system in this country. This system is supposed to always make things better and always do right by us. But that doesn't always happen and we are bitterly disappointed when it doesn't. On top of that, people all too often feel dehumanized in the process—regarded as mere numbers, and valued largely for the amount of insurance coverage they bring to the table. This is why a good insurance agent can be such an important part of your health care team and why you should review your policies regularly, as they can become outdated as your needs change with age.

THE RIGHT APPROACH TO CRISIS CARE

You absolutely need to research health insurance policies and find one that fits you and your family. It is important to have crisis coverage in place. You also need to work with the system, as it currently is—not as you want it to be. Have faith in consumer demand and expect to see the system change over time. Most importantly, accept responsibility for your own health care. You are ultimately responsible for your own health. This means staying informed and educating yourself, especially in times of a crisis. You want the best doctors and the best health care providers on your team.

When you consult with your doctor, truly *consult* with your doctor. This means asking for a meeting with your physician in his or her office prior to an examination—whenever you need to discuss anything substantial. You want your doctor to get to know you as a person. Also, go to the meeting prepared. Do some background reading beforehand. For example, let's say you are a woman in her reproductive years and are starting to experience spotting mid-cycle. Research online and look into some of the causes. Use the Internet, along with your inner guidance, to assist you in understanding your problem so that you can be a part of the solution.

Or, say you are having trouble conceiving. You aren't experiencing any other symptoms or concerns, except that you are under a lot of stress at work. Although you know that stress is a common occurrence, your intuition is telling you that it may be interfering with your ability to conceive.

If ever you are faced with a serious crisis, do your homework. Doctors are not gods; they are human beings just like you and me who happen to have an expertise in a given area. Every doctor or specialist you see might give you a different opinion, and there are numerous noninvasive options available today for you to explore. Many procedures that were written off as quackery by the political and financial powers such as acupuncture, chiropractic, and naturopathy are now mainstream and widely accepted.

Take acupuncture for example. Acupuncture is an ancient Chinese medicine treatment that has been used in the United States for around 30 years. Acupuncture involves the painless but strategic placement of tiny needles in a gridlike pattern across the body from head to toe. Acupuncture has been proven effective in assisting a wide variety of maladies, including infertility, tension headaches, asthma, pelvic pain from pregnancy, fibromyalgia, and the side effects from cancer treatments. Acupuncture appears to be growing in popularity even though it defies explanation by Western medical standards. A 2002 National Health Interview Survey indicated that 8.2 million Americans had used acupuncture. Acupuncture is believed to adjust the body's tissues, nerves, and hormones and is now approved by the National Institute of Health (NIH) and World Health Organization for treatment for certain conditions. It is a great crisis care alternative.

Maintaining your health—day to day—will strengthen your inner guidance system. And your own inner guidance will be your best ally in your quest to remain healthy as you age and postpone any crisis for as long as possible. So start by looking in a mirror. Turn and look at the curvature of your spine. Are you standing up as straight as you once did, or are you starting to slouch? Whose responsibility is this? Is your heart growing healthier and stronger as time goes by? Or is it weaker? Your health is ultimately your responsibility—not your doctor's, and certainly not your insurer's.

> **Centenarian Secret** Think of your health insurance along the same lines as homeowner's insurance. You don't have homeowner's insurance to keep your carpets clean or wipe your counters. You are responsible for these things. You are covered in case of a crisis. Day to day, you must maintain your home to keep it looking good and to prevent it from deteriorating. Your health requires the same day-to-day maintenance from you.

Don't confuse crisis care with health care. For example, if every time you have the sniffles you take an antibiotic because you believe that antibiotics will help your sniffles, you are setting your immune system up for failure. Hospitals are filled with super bugs, or antibiotic resistant bacteria. They are prolonging patient stays, increasing medical fees, and even leading to some early deaths—all because of the overuse of antibiotics. Be careful of biased science that sells a procedure. Do your homework and really learn to trust yourself.

OPTIONS
There are so many self-care and health care options out there today and the choices can be overwhelming. Where should you begin?

► **LIVE LONG AND STRONG EXERCISE**
The proactive steps I should take to avoid possible crisis care are:

1. _____
2. _____
3. _____
4. _____
5. _____

Recently a very prominent member of the community where I live had an unexpected heart attack. It became a wakeup call for him and he made the commitment to change his life. His crisis was a motivator for him. It also became a quality-of-life motivator for hundreds of other people in the community. Every type of doctor in town—from the cardiologist and internist to the chiropractor and the dentists—ended up with bookings from this one incident. People had been putting off important health care screenings. Gym memberships increased too, and heart-rate-monitor sales took a leap. Don't wait for a crisis to motivate you. Choose quality of life motivation instead, and make it your lifestyle.

Trust yourself. With everything we have discussed so far, where do you think you should begin? Do you have someone in your life whose health you would like to model? Ask for a recommendation of their providers. Interview a naturopath, a chiropractor, a general practitioner, or a cardiologist. Attend a lecture, listen to an audio, and educate yourself. Begin your discussions with a personal trainer or a nutritionist. Look into a new bed or a safer chair. Start shopping around and make a commitment that gets you in the self-care, health care game.

At some point in your life you are going to make this choice. I hope you make yours because you want to, and not because you have no choice. Let's get our priorities straight so we can all enjoy the 100-Year Lifestyle we desire with the quality of life we deserve.

THE 100-YEAR LIFESTYLE
ACTION PLAN FOR LASTING CHANGE

1. *Choose your own hierarchy.*
   If your Health Care Hierarchy has been crisis motivated and you have been on a crisis roller coaster, make self-care a priority, and get yourself on track. Decide which self-care strategies are the most appealing to you and begin to make them a part of your lifestyle, one day at a time, one choice at a time.

2. *Remember Change Principle Number 1: Change is easy—thinking about change is hard.*

It's time to make the changes you know you need to make. Stop thinking and take your first action step. Go for a walk, join a gym, set an appointment with a personal trainer, a chiropractor, or a cardiologist. Pick up the phone now and make the call. Don't put it off until a crisis.

3. *Trust yourself.*
   You know what you need to do first. Trust yourself and follow your instincts. Get on the path and stay on your path with Change Principle Number 2, and make every choice count.

4. *Educate yourself.*
   Become an expert in your ideal 100-Year Lifestyle by reading about all of the things that matter to your health so that you can become well informed and support yourself in achieving your goals. You will also be better equipped to handle any crisis that might occur if you have prepared yourself through this educational process.

5. *Build a team.*
   Build the ideal self-care, health care, and crisis care team. You probably have many of these relationships already established, and there may be some that you need to add. Do your homework. Ask your family, friends, and neighbors about their "team members" and make the appropriate appointments. Meet your team and begin implementing the game plan that you know will make a difference for you.

6. *Enjoy the journey.*
   This educational process can be fun and exciting. Your mind will begin to feel younger and your body will also, with each commitment you make.

7. *Bring a friend along for the ride.*
   Nobody wants to be alone while traveling the path to 100. Share this process with others now so that you can enjoy the journey together for 100 years and beyond. Visit *www.100yearlifestyle.com* and join the club.

PART 5

Creating the **Ideal Environment** You Can **Enjoy for 100 Years**

It's about the journey.

CHAPTER 11
ENJOY YOUR ENVIRONMENT AND MAKE THE MOST OF YOUR JOURNEY

If you are going to live an active, healthy quality of life to 100, your environment will play a key role in whether or not you enjoy the journey.

LASTING CHANGE REQUIRES CHANGING YOUR ENVIRONMENT.

The truth is that the 100-Year Lifestyle is not just about getting to 100 at all. It's not just about running a marathon to 100 and then collapsing at the finish line. It is actually more about the journey. It is not just about a quantity of years. It is about the quality of the quantity of years that you live, so that whether you make it to 80, 90, 100, or 110, you make the most of every one of them along the way. The environments you create—both the internal environment within your mind and body and the external environment where you live, work, and play—will have a lot to do with how much you enjoy your journey.

Centenarian Secret   Here is an important question to ask yourself that is a key to you making the most of your 100-Year Lifestyle. How much fun are you having?

Close your eyes after you finish this paragraph and perform this visualization with me. Describe and visualize your ideal environment. Begin with yourself: your ideal health, energy, and shape. Visualize the inner peace and personal confidence that you want. Picture yourself using your creativity and talents. Imagine using those talents to achieve mastery over something that can sustain you—for the rest of your life. Maybe you have a love of words and communication. Imagine using that skill to help others achieve clarity in the personal and professional connections they make. Or maybe you "communicate" with your hands—you love to paint or draw. Imagine drawing on and cultivating those talents professionally.

What's interesting is that when you define your ideal living environment, you will often see a pattern emerge along your family tree. One woman I came across in my travels started a new career in pottery in her forties and later discovered that a grandfather and great-grandfather were also potters—and pretty famous ones at that. You will find the greatest fulfillment when you can draw on your innate talents throughout your life. So imagine the rest of your 100 years with this in mind. Describe your ideal living environment.

Now describe your ideal external environment. Really get into the visualization so you can experience it with all of your senses. See the colors of your ideal environment, your home, your car, your office, and your vacations. What are the things that you would be doing to enjoy each day to the fullest? What are some outrageous goals you would like to achieve? Is your environment filled with trees, an ocean, lake, or river? Does it include the mountains? How are you accepted for your work? How much fun are you having and what is making life fun?

Now that you've gone through this experience and you have opened your eyes, answer this question: Are you living your ideal 100-Year Lifestyle? Is your current environment one that you can enjoy for the balance of your years? Is it a good starting point? If yes, what a fabulous foundation you have to build on. If not, get excited about the transition from where you are to where you want to be, and get ready to enjoy the journey.

There are three aspects of your environment that are important to consider in relation to creating your ideal 100-Year Lifestyle:

1. *Your inner environment.* Create a compelling vision for the rest of your life and develop the mindset to make it happen. It's got to come from you.

2. *Your external environment.* Live, work, and play in the ideal environment that resonates with your innate intelligence. Once you have the clarity, you can create and manifest your ideal environment. Sometimes this will happen quickly and sometimes slowly. The key is to move in the right direction, toward what you really want, one choice at a time. This will align your internal and external environments. Also, place yourself in external environments that feed your internal creativity. It is a cycle that continues to build your ideal 100-Year Lifestyle.

3. *Congruency between your internal and external environments, which keeps conflicts away.* Congruence between your words and your actions is powerful. Many people call it walking the talk. People who walk the talk have an inner strength regardless of their size, strength, or age. Their integrity shines through. They have a presence about them that is appealing and attractive.

The relationship between your internal environment and your external environment is crucial to a healthy, passionate, prosperous life.

Your internal environment is the one between your two ears, and the one within your skin. It is your mind, body, and spirit. You are going to be the one that has to develop the vision for your life. If someone else does it for you, you will be living somebody else's 100-Year Lifestyle and not your own. The stress of this will cause an implosion and can eventually lead to all types of challenges.

I remember hearing a speaker at a recent seminar talking about health and wellness. This particular speaker, while passionate and intense in his presentation and delivery, was 50 pounds overweight and looked stressed out of his mind. At the beginning of his presentation, the room was full. The topic was compelling. The message in the paragraph immediately following the title of his talk was very well written and designed to attract a lot of listeners—and it did.

As the speaker began to rant and rave, people began to slowly leave the room. By the end of the talk, there were only about half of the people left in the room. The mixed message between his words and his being spoke volumes to the audience and drove them away, even though his message was compelling. This is the effect of incongruence in a speaker setting, and this is also the effect of incongruence in life.

I have seen incongruence between a person's internal and external environments cause frustration to them in so many ways, costing them money, love, and health to name a few. A few years ago I went to visit one of my clients who was a family practice doctor. He wanted his practice to be filled with a lot of kids and families. He had taken all the extra training necessary to develop his skills in this area. He wanted to educate families to raise healthy, drug-free kids. This doctor had the financial backing of his parents, who wanted him to have the nicest office on the planet. They put him through school, found his location, and built one of the most beautiful offices I have ever seen. It was a great external environment.

Unfortunately for this inexperienced doctor, they also decorated the office like his grandmother's living room. You know what I mean, the kind where everything is so perfect that you are afraid to leave a footprint on the carpet, a fingerprint on the counter, or a butt print on the couch. No matter how hard this doctor tried to attract families to his practice for care, he couldn't do it. People were afraid they would mess up his beautiful space. It was not the ideal external environment for families, even though in his heart, that is what he wanted to attract. This incongruence cost him dearly until he finally changed his environment.

At first he resisted these changes that I knew he needed to make. He argued about why he couldn't make the changes. Finally I was able to convince him to make some external changes that were more congruent with his internal vision for his practice, and he immediately became more magnetic to kids and families.

He changed the coffee table from sharp, pointy edge glass to rounded corners with wood. He added some stuffed animals and a video game to his reception area. He put some family friendly posters up. These subtle changes to his external environment, which were congruent with his internal environment, turned his practice around overnight.

We've spent so much time on giving you the health and energy to live a long healthy life. Now let's take the steps to fully enjoy the journey every step of the way.

CHAPTER 12
CREATING YOUR IDEAL ENVIRONMENT WHEREVER YOU GO

W e have already spent quite a bit of time on your internal environment. We've worked a lot on getting your mindset excited about the opportunities that come with an extended life span and have given you strategies to maintain youthful energy. We've hopefully gotten you to eliminate destructive patterns that are taking years off your life and helped you to establish a health care plan.

Now it's time to create the vision for your extended life so that the rest of your life is exciting, inspiring, and one that you would want to live, remembering Change Principle Number 3: Approach change with your ideal 100-Year Lifestyle in mind. The fact is that if you do not have a vision for your life with exciting new goals to achieve and things to accomplish, then you are going to have to create it. The more clearly you can visualize it, the more likely you will be able to transition to it immediately or over time, and the more fun the rest of your life will be. What is your ideal lifestyle? The one you would like to live? If you do not develop a clear vision to construct your future, you will end up reconstructing your past over and over again.

One of the challenges of today's centenarians has been a lack of vision for their later years. Once they retire they spend their days watching the news and checking the mail. There are so many exciting options when you continue to set new goals, challenge yourself, and explore the world. It's your decision, and you are the one who is going to have to make it happen.

Centenarian Secret You can either construct your future, or you can continue to reconstruct the past. But you can't do both at the same time. You have to choose.

There is an old saying in the consulting world that goes something like this: Take a successful business owner and put him or her in a failing business and they will turn that business around and make it successful. On the other hand, if you take the owner of a failing business and put him or her in a successful one, it won't be too long before they turn that business around, and drive it into the ground as well. I have seen many doctors do this to their practices. I have seen numerous patients do this also. They moved into my town and they unconsciously re-created their life exactly as it was in the previous location. You are at the perfect starting place to set up things exactly as you want if you are willing to change your mind and create a compelling vision for your future.

And as you transition yourself with Change Principle Number 2, make sure you acknowledge your progress along the way, because changing your environment is a process that takes time— unless you were like me and were forced there by a crisis.

This happened to me in 1994, a time when I wanted to make a lot of changes in my life. I was in my early thirties, I had a young family, I had a growing practice, and I was working only 20 miles from home, but the commuter traffic kept me in the car much more than I wanted.

The strain of trying to make everything work was affecting my work life and my family life. I wanted to move my office closer to home. However, my office was in a great location—on Peachtree Road in Buckhead, which is an affluent and very commercial part of Atlanta—and I was reluctant to make the change. I had a terrific practice and I was established there. Fear of the unknown kept me stuck in place. I didn't know if my clients would follow me to a new location and if I could build an equally successful practice in another part of town. I also knew that I wanted to change the environment of that office. It had become stifling because my practice had grown so much that the original layout of the office had created some capacity issues and flow problems as we grew. People had to wait for a longer period of time than they really should have, and all of this was due to the environment.

So I stayed stuck for a while. Eventually it took a crisis for me to make the changes I knew I needed to make. The crisis came in the form of a little old lady who lost control of her car in the parking lot, stepped on the gas instead of the brakes, and plowed her car right through the center of my office at 40 miles per hour. Can you imagine that? I had the first drive-through chiropractic office in history. Thank God this happened just before my busiest time with patients, so there were only a few people in the office. Initially I was really traumatized. I wasn't thinking clearly, I didn't know what to do, and I was having some post-traumatic stress. My internal environment was not functioning in a healthy way. All I could see was the destruction in my external environment. It was like I had blinders on that blocked out the possibilities that existed from the destruction.

Around a week later, with the help of my wife and some good friends and family members, I realized that I needed to start thinking about the situation differently. Yes, I had this destruction happening that needed to be cleaned up. Yes, I had this challenge and I began to realize internally that I could either continue to play the victim or I could shift my environment. There were so many changes that I had been wanting to make to the layout of the office so it would flow better. Finally, I decided to view the crisis as an opportunity to make the changes that I had wanted to make for a long time. I began to look for the good and seek out the opportunities that were delivered by this angel. What happened then was miraculous.

I started to get excited about the opportunity to re-create my vision. I realized now, because of the accident, I could do it and save the demolition costs. It was an opportunity to set up the office to help more people. Also, I decided that maybe this was the time to move and open a second office. I began to drive around my home neighborhood and see if there were any new office locations that were available. The ideal space that I had been looking at within a mile of my house became available that day. I got psyched, and within two months, I opened a new office right where I wanted to be. The opportunity was right there but I wouldn't have seen it if I wasn't willing to change my mind about things and open up to acting on my vision and building a compelling future. I learned to package my thoughts differently. I learned to turn the crisis into an opportunity.

GET CREATIVE AND USE SOME DIFFERENT LOBULES OF YOUR BRAIN

The opportunity that we all have with longevity is incredible. We have the chance to learn—and to use what we learn over time to continue to build our lives. What a great gift. This is what I call "a lobule jump," referring to the different parts of the brain (called *lobules*) we use to perform certain tasks and solve problems. Rather than getting caught up in a certain thought pattern, which can lead to overanalyzing and paralysis of analysis, you can open up your mind to see things differently by shifting to a different lobule of your brain.

Very often we get stuck seeing things a certain way rather than using our entire mind to see all sides. Like a holograph that changes pictures when you change your angle, so does nearly every situation that relates to your environment—you've just got to be willing to stretch your brain to see things differently.

When was the last time you looked at a picture of a brain? Isn't it amazing that this mass of matter, when animated with life, can run your entire body, adapt you to your environment, and originate thought? In computer scans you can see these lobules light up when they process information. For instance, the right lobule may activate when the brain is reading or interpreting language and the left side when you are translating complex mathematics or conducting three-dimensional visualization.

In fact, researchers performing postmortem studies on the brain of Albert Einstein found that his left inferior parietal lobules were larger than in most humans. The study, published in the *Lancet* in 1999, postulated that both Einstein's left lobe (the one responsible for complex mathematic calculations and spatial reasoning) and the right one might have expanded early in his prenatal development. You can make a lobule jump by asking different questions and taking new actions based on the new answers.

I remember working with a patient who was having a lot of trouble with her spine. She was in a really stressful job and was sitting around ten hours a day. She would then go home and wouldn't eat properly or exercise, and just crash on the couch and sit there until bedtime. She loved her chiropractic care because she always felt better when she got adjusted, but she would continually re-create her problems by the way she was living her life.

Every other aspect of her environment—from the way she thought, sat, and ate, to the way she structured her day—was destructive. I spoke with her about changing her internal environment—from the way she thought to the way she ate to the way she exercised. On top of that, I also advised her on ways to change her external environment—from where she ate to where she shopped to how she spent her day.

Changing her environment, both internal and external, was important for producing lasting change to her quality of life. It was amazing because by making these changes, she was able to end the destructive patterns that held her back. She was able to take her health to the next level, and this began to spill over into the rest of her life.

Centenarian Secret   Create a compelling vision for the rest of your life. What do you want to accomplish? What goals do you want to achieve? What experiences would you like to explore? Don't get stuck operating in only one part of your brain when approaching challenges and opportunities. Make a lobule jump to move past negative self-perceptions or disempowering thoughts. By staying in the same part of the brain instead of expanding into other lobules, you may create the same scenarios over and over again.

Lobule jumping is about opening up opportunities and possibilities and moving past mental obstacles. If you keep doing the same thing you always do, you're going to keep getting the same thing you always get. The easiest way to make a lobule jump is to simply take action. That may simply mean accepting the situation at first, and then taking appropriate action.

What does this look like? Well, I think of my wife's grandfather, Hyman Sperling.

"Papa Hy" turns 100 this year. He's a special man and very dear to our family. In 1992, he lost his house during a hurricane. He was in his mid-eighties and had to rebuild his life from scratch. I asked him about it recently. "What is there to talk about?" he said. "It was a hurricane; it destroyed the house, the furniture, and everything in it. All we salvaged were some clothes that we wore. That's all." There was no pity, no analysis—although, maybe a touch of anger. The key was that he took action. "There was an apartment available in Coral Springs. We took it. I think it was $700 a month and we had to pay a three-month advance. We paid around $3,500 and we lived there for six weeks. So we got out of there and bought an apartment in Palm Springs and that is where I'm living now."

In times of crisis, always think Change Principle Number 2: Think progress, not perfection.

CHANGE THE WAY YOU THINK

You can change your life by changing the way you think. By using different pathways and asking new questions, you can find exciting solutions.

The types of questions on the facing page open you up to greater possibilities that will invite exciting opportunities into your extended life. By acting on one or two of these at a time you will begin to attract the clarity that helps you create the environment you will enjoy for a lifetime. These are much better questions than . . . What's wrong with me? Why am I such an idiot? Why can't I reach my goals? Why bother, I am already 60 years old?

▶ LIVE LONG AND STRONG EXERCISE

Start lighting up new lobules of your brain to create a life without limits by asking these core questions:

- » How can I be more effective in my life?
- » What are the core values that I want to base my life on?
- » Who can be my mentor and help me achieve my goals?
- » How can I be a better professional?
- » What would make me a better listener?
- » Who do I need to learn from to do my job better?
- » How can I make myself heard in a positive way?
- » What habit can I commit to that will change my life for the better?
- » What commitments will make me a healthier person?
- » What can I accept about my past that will enable me to move forward?
- » Who can I forgive today so that I can let go and live my life?
- » What resources are available to me?
- » What do I really want?
- » Where do I want to live?
- » What colors make me feel happy inside and would improve my environment?
- » What changes can I make to my home to make it more enjoyable?
- » What do I want my finances to be like in a year?
- » What choices do I need to make to achieve that goal?
- » What do I want from my life partner that I am not getting right now?
- » How can I ask for it so that I am more likely to receive it?
- » What do I need to give in order to have my partner feel secure?
- » How can I use my talents and passions to earn extra money?

Asking new and better questions will bring you answers that support your ideal 100-Year Lifestyle.

Thoughts can keep you in destructive patterns. Changing your thoughts about things can propel you into a human potential pattern that attracts your ideal 100-Year Lifestyle to you magnetically. Remember Change Principle Number 1: Change is easy—thinking about change is hard. Dare yourself to dream and then make your dreams come true. After all, you get to start fresh with decades of experience under your belt. What an opportunity if you are willing to see it this way.

Think about the thoughts and attitudes you bring to every situation. Does the party get going when you get there or does it fall apart? Does a room feel more comfortable when you are there or do you create stress? Do you meet nice people wherever you go, or do you always find the jerk in the crowd? Do you find a financial opportunity in every situation? The one commonality in every environment you enter is you. You are going to take yourself with you wherever you go. Rather than judge yourself, you have an opportunity to look at the results you are creating and decide if you like them. If you don't like them, you can decide whether you want to change them—by changing your views and your vision. A change in your environment must begin with you.

ACCEPTING OUR CURRENT ENVIRONMENT

Dr. C is one of my clients who has an office in Virginia. Since mastering many of these 100-Year Lifestyle principles his patient base has grown dramatically, his income has nearly tripled, and he is having more fun than ever in his practice and his life. In the early stages of his training, he was an extremely stressed-out doctor. Every time one of his patients didn't do exactly what he wanted them to do, he would get severely stressed out. During the summer when most of his clients were on vacation, he'd get mad that they would miss their appointments. His stress level was so high that he literally drove away close to 20 employees in three years. He was so busy trying to control everything that he was missing a terrific opportunity: to take a much-needed break.

One day we were on the phone, and I asked him to stand up. Once he got up, I asked him to squat down as low as he could go, and then jump up as high as he possibly could. I told him not to stop until he reached the clouds. He chuckled and didn't even try to jump. When I asked him why he was laughing, he told me that my request was ridiculous. I said, "I know it is ridiculous, but go ahead and do it anyway." Jump up and touch the clouds.

He jumped and obviously within one second, his feet were back on the ground. When I asked him why he came back to the ground, he laughed again and said, "gravity."

"Are you angry at gravity?" I asked him. He said, "Of course not. I can't control the forces of gravity."

Trying to control all of the things that are out of your control is like trying to control gravity. Accepting the things that are out of your control and facing the reality of them will open the door to exciting opportunities. This simple conversation was life changing to him because now, instead of getting angry when his entire town is on vacation, he vacations during that time himself. He has turned it into great play time. He gets the rest, pleasure, and enjoyment of wonderful vacations without losing any real productivity, and he is much more energized and focused when he returns to work. The quality of the care he provides has improved dramatically because he is well rested and able to give his all to his patients. What used to be a very difficult and challenging time for him has turned into a great opportunity because he was willing to change his view of the situation. He is using a different lobule.

Part of our internal struggle is that we grow up learning to think about things a certain way. We cling to a lot of our early beliefs even when it is no longer in our best interest to do so. I have a client, a highly successful businessperson with a family of her own, who is now caring for her ailing mother. Unfortunately, her mother is overly critical of her. There is a part of this woman that still values her mother's opinion more than her own. I said to her, "You are 50 years old. At some point, you are going to have

Neal and Lori Plasker

"My cousin Neal is an incredible man who just a few years ago lost his wife to cancer after a grueling 11-year battle. During that time he stood by her side with first-class integrity and commitment.

Initially when Barbara was diagnosed with lung cancer—a very rare form—the only hope for her was going to be a double lung transplant operation. They did all the necessary preparation and made arrangements to be on-call so Barbara could receive her new lungs. Finally the day came, and they flew to Birmingham for the surgery.

Lisa and I drove over to support them, as did several of our other family members. The surgery was a success. Barbara went through some intense rehabilitation and after several months was able to begin to enjoy her life again. She and Neal spent time with the kids and over the next few years, they got to see their youngest son get bar mitzvahed and their daughter get married, and attend several family members' high school and college graduations.

Ultimately, in August 2004, the cancer got the best of Barbara and the last few years of the battle were emotionally and physically exhausting for everyone in the family. Neal stood by Barbara's side and did his best to ease her suffering. His loyalty and commitment to her was a constant source of strength to the entire family.

Several months after Barbara's passing, Neal decided that he was still alive, and after many years of making the most of his life under difficult circumstances—which in my heart was a key to Barbara surviving so long—he decided he was ready to live life to the fullest, and he was open to finding love again. If there was anyone who deserved it, it was Neal. Several months later, he met a woman named Lori. They were a match.

Lori has her own story. She had a long but challenging marriage, which produced two beautiful children. Eventually, she found the courage to get a divorce. She continued to raise her daughters and got used to living on her own. Several years later, on her fiftieth birthday, she blew out the candles on her cake surrounded by close family and friends. Her life was full and good. She had completely healed from her divorce and she realized that she was deeply content and happy.

Soon afterward, a friend asked Lori about setting her up on a blind date. That man was Neal. Lori knew of Neal and had heard he was a good man. She remembers being very nervous on their first date. On their second date, Neal touched Lori's shoulder. Instantly Lori felt for the first time in a very long time that she was "home." Neal and Lori fell in love, got married, and are now building an incredible life together. They are doing a fabulous job blending their two families—Neal, with his three children, son-in-law, and new grandchild, and Lori, with her two daughters. They are committed to creating and sharing lots of great times and they have expanded their rock solid support system.

Neal and Lori have found true love after the age of 50. With a little luck and the principles of the 100-Year Lifestyle on their side, Neal, who is now 52, and Lori, who is 51, could celebrate their silver, even a golden anniversary together, even though they are starting their journey together during midlife."

to decide that your mother's opinion is just her opinion and you are entitled to one too. You have to decide if your opinion is the same as your mother's or father's, or if it is going to be different. My opinion is that you're a really good person, a really talented person, and a really successful person."

Which opinion do you choose to believe? Which one do you want to nurture for the rest of your life? The one that says you can have fun and enjoy an active, healthy, prosperous life for 100 years and beyond? Or the one that says you are already old, getting older by the second, and you will end up in a nursing home? Why do we make the negative more important than the positive and exciting? What an unnecessary energy drain that stifles our environment and keeps us from seeing all the opportunities that are right under our noses.

Instead, we should place our energy and focus on the compelling vision we wish to create as we customize our ideal 100-Year Lifestyle.

THE ISSUE ABOUT OUR ISSUES

We all have issues. I've learned this from taking care of thousands of patients from all walks of life. I've taken care of celebrities, royalty, professional athletes, and multimillionaires as well as many ordinary people. I've taken care of healthy people who were committed to a wellness lifestyle. I've also taken care of people who were really sick and suffering. It is amazing how different people respond to their issues, and we all have them—all of us.

The question you have to ask yourself as you change your internal environment is: Do you want to make your issues your life? Or do you want to make your life your life? The people who are having the most fun—and are also the most successful at reaching their goals and achieving balance—are the ones who manage their issues while they live their ideal life. They make their life more important than their issues. They are able to keep things in a perspective that makes inner peace, fulfillment, and happiness more important than their challenges.

Developing a compelling vision for your 100-Year Lifestyle is crucial to your long-term success, health, and happiness and shifts your energy off your issues. Not doing this has been one of the biggest challenges for many of our current seniors and centenarians. Because they didn't know they were going to live as long as they have, many of them have developed destructive, survival, or complacent thought patterns that are causing them to deteriorate way before they should.

Changing your view of longevity from a 60- or 70-year lifestyle to a 100-Year Lifestyle changes the way you view your life. Develop a vision for your extended life and then change your external environment to match.

When my father got sick with Alzheimer's, everyone in my family was in denial about his condition. My mother, on the other hand, because she lived with him every day, knew that his condition was progressing rapidly. Her ability to accept her situation enabled her to make the best choices to deal with her issues, and live her life. She handles her issues and my dad's issues while she also lives her life.

While we all watched him deteriorate, we also watched her take the lead on the action steps necessary that, in the long run, were the best for him and the best for her—even though those decisions were difficult ones. What was amazing to me was that during this process, she continued to try and live her best life and make choices that were through progress, not perfection, taking her down the best road for all of us who were involved.

My father is now in a home and my mother holds a position that enables her to use her skills as an adult educator. She is making a difference for others and helping people reach their full potential, which is her primary purpose in life. She transitioned from a high-stress intense commute that would have kept her away from my dad, to now working within one minute of where my father lives. She sees him nearly every day. She has remained loyal and loving to him after 45 years of marriage and through his illness, while using her talents to make a difference as an educator—creating programs for seniors that improve their quality of life.

Centenarian Secret   To be able to accept your current situation while you also remain committed to creating your compelling future, one choice at a time, is a tremendous skill to develop.

At some of our seminars, we do a hiking session that is all about personal breakthroughs. At one event in particular, I remember going for a walk with a group of seminar attendees at Stone Mountain Park just outside of Atlanta. We climbed up Stone Mountain and when we reached the top, we could see for miles. The landscape was illuminated at certain angles by thousands of homes. Their rooftops penetrated the sky at all different heights. I realized that day that inside every one of those buildings was a reality, a vision, a way of viewing the world that differed in big or small ways from my own as well as from each other. Each reality was defined not only by a unique set of values, experiences, and ambitions, but also by a unique approach to life.

It became clear to me that day, that it is generally more important what happens inside the four walls of each house than outside. What the owner of each house sees from the inside is the only thing he or she can manifest on the outside.

Think about what happens at seven in the morning when the multimillionaire and the construction worker wake up and go to work each day. Both are honorable people with different experiences and views of the world. They breathe the same air, drink the same water, and live in the same state. Because they have different visions for their life, they manifest different results in their life.

How about two people in different homes that both make $50,000 a year, and one is in debt up to his eyeballs and one is saving money every month. Depending on the vision you see for your life, you will manifest what your mind can see. The internal environment you choose to see will take you as far as you are willing to go. Why not choose to see your ideal 100-Year Lifestyle?

TAP INTO YOUR CREATIVITY

You have to be able to see your life as active, healthy, prosperous, and fun for 100 years in order to create a vision that is compelling. What would be a really exciting and fun life to live for the next 50 years? Begin to talk about it with your life partner, your friends, and your colleagues. Start to voice your vision and bring it into your consciousness. Putting words to it and continuing a dialogue will help you gain the clarity you need to attract the resources, people, and things you need to transition yourself from your current environment to your new one.

We've all heard of the expression "think outside the box." This is lobule jumping. This is an important part of changing your internal and external environment. Drive around different neighborhoods and office parks and look at the various signs, houses, cars, and everything related to environments that are different from yours, but ones you would like to experience. Begin to ask yourself, how do these people think that is different from the way I think?

Start asking questions that open your mind to being able to create a new experience for yourself. Open up to these new possibilities and begin to envision how you can change your environment and make it ideal.

Don't just ask you, however; get to know people who can be mentors for you at your stage of life. One thing I have learned about people who are winning in life is that they are usually very willing to help out others who are seriously committed to changing their lives. It's all about intent and the reasons behind your motivation. Widen your scope—think outside of yourself and find a greater purpose—and like the magnets of Change Principle Number 1, you will begin to attract more good things with ease. Narrowing the scope of your intent and being self-righteous and self-centered will repel new and exciting opportunities that are right under your nose. Think about a camera lens. A wide-angle lens expands your field of vision. Be willing to change your internal environment and look through a bigger and broader lens.

Think like a champion. List five key attitudes that you can cultivate immediately to attract your ideal 100-Year Lifestyle:

1. _____
   _____

2. _____
   _____

3. _____
   _____

4. _____
   _____

5. _____
   _____

What are five activities that you can do to cultivate those attitudes? Examples are finding a coach or a mentor, forming a mastermind group with high-achieving people who are embracing these 100-Year Lifestyle concepts, joining a neighborhood association and getting involved in activities that improve your community, attending a seminar, participating in a community-development project through work, or joining a civic organization.

1. _____
   _____

2. _____
   _____

3. _____
   _____

4. _____
   _____

5. _____
   _____

List at least ten goals that would be exciting to achieve over the next decade.

1. _____
2. _____
3. _____
4. _____
5. _____
6. _____
7. _____
8. _____
9. _____
10. _____

List at least ten things you would absolutely love to do before you turn 100. If you want to list 100 things, go for it. I encourage you to do this. Start a journal and call it 100-year goals and then fill it up.

1. _____
2. _____
3. _____
4. _____
5. _____
6. _____
7. _____
8. _____
9. _____
10. _____

CHAPTER 13
BALANCING YOUR INTERNAL AND EXTERNAL ENVIRONMENTS

This chapter was the hardest chapter in the book for me to write. When I initially went through the manuscript, I completed every chapter and was ecstatic about them. When I got to this chapter, I wrote a fragmented outline and could not really get the flow going. No matter how hard I tried, I got stuck. I flew through the rest of the book and created what I believed was very compelling, life-changing content. But then I had to go back to this one.

It drove me crazy that I could not get this chapter done, knowing how important environment is to the 100-Year Lifestyle.

Finally I realized what the problem was. My external environment was stagnant. It was stifling me. It was cluttered. It wasn't fresh. It had an accumulation of stuff that was no longer significant to me and was just taking up space. There were old clothes stuffed in our closets that were out of style and didn't fit right anymore. There were old books, lots of them, filling up shelves, desktops, and floors. There were numerous repairs that needed to be made to the house, along with several unfinished projects. We had been talking about moving for the last few years and left our environment in limbo, along with this chapter. Wouldn't you know I had to fix my own external environment before I could finish.

I declared a family workday and Lisa, the kids, and I went on a cleansing binge. We freed up the space—throwing out 100 big bags of garbage, giving away 20 bags of clothes, and 11 boxes of books to charity.

After that, this chapter came together for me instantly on the day that I declared our family workday and committed to cleansing our environment. Change really is much easier than thinking about change.

Is your environment stifling to you? Or is it the one that you can enjoy for the balance of your years? Do you have 50 incomplete projects laying around? How are they impacting your energy? Are you feeling stuck?

Take action immediately by changing your external environment. Start with where you are and begin to cleanse. Cleaning up your environment opens up the space for new, exciting ideas and opportunities that will free your creative spirit and bring freshness into your life.

For my family, this cleansing has opened up a lot of exciting opportunities for all of us. Our vision for our life and environment

▶ **LIVE LONG AND STRONG EXERCISE**

Define your ideal home environment:

_____

What is currently missing from this environment that you would like to add?

_____

Define your ideal work environment:

_____

What is currently missing from this environment that you would like to add?

_____

What changes do you need to make to create the ideal environment you can enjoy for 100 years?

_____

What unfinished projects do you need to complete?

_____

▶ LIVING THE 100-YEAR LIFESTYLE:
Jon Butcher

Jon Butcher, chairman of the Precious Moments Family of Companies and cofounder of the Creating Wellness Alliance, and creator of mylifebook.com, offers this story of creating an environment to match his 100-Year Lifestyle.

"When my wife and I sat down to design our dream house, we made a conscious decision to build a home that clearly projected the values, moods, and feelings we wanted in our lives on a continuous basis. Although there were a number of key values we focused on, we defined the most important group as the "healing values" of tranquility, peacefulness, and serenity. I run a number of big businesses and life can be stressful, so we wanted to create an environment that would care for us, revive us, and allow us to recover from the day's demands. Like most people in industrialized countries, we spend 90 percent of our time indoors, so we saw a healthy building as part of our health plan—an investment in our physical and mental well-being.

We used the following recipe to achieve our goal: First, we invited nature into our home. We focused on the sight and sound of water by building small waterfalls throughout the house, so we could see and hear flowing water from just about every room. We built planters around our waterfalls so we would be surrounded by growing, living things 365 days a year. We flooded the house with natural light by utilizing skylights, windows, and sliding glass doors. We installed a music system with speakers throughout the entire house and spent many hours compiling play lists of soft, relaxing music (there is no single factor that is more important to setting a mood than music). We welcomed health and fitness into our home with a major commitment to a gym and a small spa, and designed numerous relaxation and meditation areas that melt away stress. We chose natural materials and a neutral color palette for the entire home to assure that nothing shouts for attention—and the effect is a sedate, peaceful, and calm environment. Finally, we built in two large fireplaces for warmth and comfort—and we focused on comfortable, informal furniture throughout the home.

As a couple, our commitment to our environment has kept our relationship passionate and alive, has been instrumental to the growth of my company, and has been a catalyst for me helping to transform other people's lives."

has been creatively inspired. We are more excited about enter-taining again and sharing our beautiful home with friends and family. We are more relaxed during our play time when we are at home. Our chronic stress has gone down, which has freed up energy for other things. We have opened up more vision-oriented discussions within our family about our own ideal 100-Year Lifestyle environment. Change sure is easy and thinking about change can sure be hard.

SOME WAYS TO CONTROL YOUR EXTERNAL ENVIRONMENT

One way of reducing stress caused by your environment is to get in the habit of completing activities that you begin. I have a good friend who has ten major projects going on at once in his home and it is really causing a lot of stress to his family. Loose ends can make you lose your mind.

Also, stimulate your environment with music and spend less time in front of the television. With digital video recorders it is so easy and inexpensive these days to filter through the television muck and fill your life with the few shows that are important to you. Of course, you can also watch them at a time that is con-venient for you, rather than rushing to catch your favorite show before it starts. In today's day and age, television begins when you want it to and you can turn it off whenever you want also.

Further, make sure your environment is in line with your per-sonality. When Lisa and I moved into our first home, we invested a lot of money to decorate it. We were young and excited, and we decided on a style that was exactly like our parents' style. While the décor was first-class and nice, we realized a few months later that while it was beautiful, it wasn't our style. As you gain matu-rity—which is the beauty of being able to begin life again with 40, 50, or 60 years' experience—you really begin to connect with your own style. From the clothes you wear to the colors in your home, you can totally change the look and feel of your life by cul-tivating a willingness to think outside your box and experiment with different styles.

Also, reconsider time that you "don't have any control over." For instance, not too long ago, one of my patients took a new job that required her to spend a total of two hours in her vehicle commuting to and from work. While the job alleviated some of her financial stress, it added to her emotional and mental stress. In fact, the aggravation and anxiety that accompanied sitting in traffic became so acute that it interfered with her ability to work once she finally got into the office.

I helped her see this new circumstance as an opportunity. I pointed out to her that an hour each way translated into ten hours a week, or 520 hours a year of time that she now had to develop her knowledge and skills in any endeavor she wishes. She can use the time to listen to self-help or motivational tapes, learn a language, hear a book on tape, or tutor herself in business or other areas of interest. Soon, she began to see this time as a resource and as an opportunity for growth. She no longer let her commute time cause her stress.

She has since quit her job and started a home-based business using her core talents and she combines them with many of the concepts she learned while commuting. What an opportunity her commute turned out to be. She stimulated her internal environment to make changes in her external environment, and you are doing the exact same thing by reading this book. You are stimulating your internal environment, which will cause you to take action and start creating your ideal 100-Year Lifestyle.

Experiences That You Give Yourself

Try changing your external environment from the drugstore to the health food store. You'd be amazed at how many millions of people who used to depend on drugs for everyday living now just choose to eat healthier, take supplements, get adjusted, and exercise regularly to ensure they are as healthy as possible. Change your environment from a fast-food restaurant to a healthy alternative. Drive to the gym instead of the mall. Rearrange your furniture. Change things up and begin to view the world a little differently to stimulate your creativity.

Destructive patterns in your environment reinforce your current life. For example, driving to the liquor store on your way home each night will ensure that you drink. Going out for ice cream every night will ensure that you continue to pack on the pounds. Replace these destructive energy patterns with new human potential patterns and support them with healthy, 100-Year Lifestyle environment choices.

This is why your shopping patterns are important. Remember, what you buy and where you buy it is important, because wherever you shop, you'll end up bringing some of those items back home. Again, a little magnetism is at play here. You can't sit on a lint-covered couch and not pick up a little lint too. Rather than trying to avoid the lint, which will ultimately be futile anyway, your best bet is to keep a clean environment.

A common mistake we make is to try to prove to ourselves that we are past our old habits by pushing ourselves back into

▶ **LIVE LONG AND STRONG EXERCISE**

Describe your ideal home environment:

_____

_____

_____

Describe your ideal work environment:

_____

_____

_____

Describe your ideal vacation environment:

_____

_____

_____

negative patterns and trying to resist them. In reality, this is neither growth nor change. It's like you've taken a vacation from the
real you. Stick to the same patterns and before you know it, you'll
be back to the same routine, suffering from the same challenges
as before. You'll know that you're really "past" something when
you have shut the door on it forever and don't feel the urge to look
back. This is a sign of real change.

Create an external environment that resonates with your
internal environment and supports your human potential pattern. Take all of your old memorabilia in your home that is no
longer relevant or supportive of the next phase of your life and
box it up. If it is relevant but a part of your history, move it to a
designated place in your home where you keep all of your past.
Designate this area as your personal museum, and fill the rest of
your environment with things that inspire your future or help
you make the most enjoyment out of the present. Do the same
thing at work by filling your environment with elements that
enhance a positive and productive attitude. When you enjoy your
space at home, at work, in your car, and in your daily activities,
you will feed the lifestyle you deserve and desire.

BE CONGRUENT INSIDE AND OUT

The key is to create an external environment that is congruent with
your internal one. This congruency will give you peace of mind,
keep you centered, and establish an environment and lifestyle that is
uniquely important to you. When your internal and external environment are not congruent, the consequences can be destructive.

I noticed an example of incongruence one day when I saw
a beautiful Mercedes convertible stopped at a traffic light with
the music blasting. At first glance I noticed the car and said to
myself, "Wow, that's a beautiful car." Then I thought to myself,
"That person must be very successful." Finally, I looked through
the window and saw a 300-pound man crammed into the driver
seat with the steering wheel pressing a two-inch indent in his
stomach. I wonder how he got in there. I wonder how he gets out.
And how on earth does he drive with the steering wheel wedged

against his bulging abdomen? This unfortunate soul is headed for a serious crisis and I'm not sure which will come first, the car accident or the heart attack. I wonder how long he will be able to enjoy that beautiful automobile.

Additional areas of incongruence can be living above your means, tolerating abusive relationships, eating healthy or starving yourself all day and binging at night, and compromising your voice by not speaking up when you know you have something valuable to say.

Congruency with your internal environment and your external one will help you create your ideal 100-Year Lifestyle and give you the inner peace to enjoy the journey every step of the way.

As you do the Live Long and Strong exercises throughout this book you will probably begin to notice a pattern of things to do that repeat themselves over and over again. This is exciting

▶ **LIVE LONG AND STRONG EXERCISE**

Identify areas of incongruence between your internal environment and your external environment:

_____

_____

_____

How are they affecting you?

_____

_____

_____

The immediate thoughts and actions you can take to create congruency are:

_____

_____

_____

because you will realize that the closer you get to your core, the simpler it is to transition to your environment and the changes that you know you need to make. Start having more fun than ever by committing to the internal and external environments that feed your mind, body, and spirit. You already know what to do. Now that you feel better, have more energy, and have begun to change your environment, let's begin to attract the right people into our lives and build on our experiences and maximize the enjoyment of the next phase of our extended lives.

CARING FOR OUR GLOBAL ENVIRONMENT

Let's spend a few minutes talking about the environment that we all share—the planet. As the world's population continues to grow, the impact of this growth is likely to catch up to us. I think again of my 300-pound friend driving the beautiful Mercedes who was busting out of his space. As the world's population grows, it is more important than ever that we live in sync with our environment and not put short-term gains ahead of our collective long-term health.

Let's be quality-of-life motivated versus crisis motivated when it comes to our natural resources. We know we all want to breathe clean air and drink clean water. We all want to enjoy the oceans, mountains, lakes, and streams. Every choice we make affects our environment—from the way we dispose of our waste products to the items we buy in the store. Green buildings are in because responsible builders are realizing that workers want to be in an environment that is healthy. And what is healthy for us is also healthy for our environment.

"Green" is predicted to be one of the growth industries in this millennium, and thank goodness. Green construction by definition is quality construction—no corners are cut, and waste is kept to a minimum. Learn about builders in your area that specialize in green building and learn about their certification and knowledge.

"Green" homes rival "smart" homes in terms of awe-inspiring features and amenities like geothermal heating and windows with photo-chromatic glazing, which grow darker to block out heat in the summer, but stay clear in winter. "You see the shift toward green through the number of green products now making their way into the marketplace," says Steven Kleber, the head of a marketing firm in Atlanta specializing in products for the home. "We've seen a change not only in terms of the sheer volume of products, but also in terms of their variation and the number of companies entering the market. Many of our best-known companies will eventually tap this market."

The key thing to remember is that you don't have to uproot your life to be green. There are a million and one little things you can start doing today to protect the environment. They include recycling, turning off lights, and installing a dehumidifier onto your central AC system to pull moisture out of the air in the summer—allowing you to cool more efficiently. If you are building a home, look into construction materials and, most importantly, builders that work in sync with the environment. Like the titration experiment we discussed in Life Changing Principle Number 2, every drop counts!

▶ **LIVE LONG AND STRONG EXERCISE**
List three things you can start doing today to live more in sync with your environment:

1. _____

_____

_____

2. _____

_____

_____

3. _____

_____

_____

THE 100-YEAR LIFESTYLE
ACTION PLAN FOR LASTING CHANGE

1. *Have gratitude and appreciate your current environment.*
Look for the good and make the most of your current environment. If you are not willing to take the time to begin constructing your future in your current environment, you will probably re-create the past in your new one if you move.

2. *Begin to develop your vision for your ideal 100-Year Lifestyle.*
Verbalize your dreams with people who are close to you, who you trust to support you in creating it. Keep a journal of the things that are important to you for your internal and external environment. Continue to define and redefine, with more and more clarity, your ideal 100-Year Lifestyle.

3. *Complete the attitudes that attract exercise.*
Begin to train yourself to think outside the box and magnetically attract what you want. Catch yourself when your thoughts move into destructive patterns and immediately shift yourself back to your ideal mindset.

4. *Let go of trying to control the things that are out of your control.*
Focus on the things that you can change. Through this acceptance and letting go process you will begin to formulate a transition strategy that will help you change your environment.

5. *Describe your ideal home and work environments.*
Identify any changes that you can immediately make to improve your environment and make it more enjoyable.

6. *Start having more fun and enjoying the journey now.*
Look for the good in every situation. Appreciate your progress and the lessons you have learned. They have set the stage for you to maximize the rest of your 100 years.

7. *Be good to the planet.*
Become environmentally conscious and encourage your family and friends to do the same. We are all in this together.

PART 6

Building a
Rock Solid
Support
System
You Can Enjoy
for 100
Years

*Nobody wants
to get to 100 alone.*

CHAPTER 14
CONNECTING WITH MULTIPLE GENERATIONS AND CIRCLES OF PEOPLE

y this stage of the game, you know what's best for your health and your environment. These are key components of enjoying a quality 100 years because nobody wants to age suffering the consequences of pain, sickness, and disease, while also living in an unpleasant environment that is out of their control. In my interviews with people all over the world, another key concern that people have about aging is loneliness.

NOBODY WANTS TO GET TO 100 ALONE

This chapter is about creating a rock solid support system that you can enjoy for 100 years. I call this the Surround Sound System of Support. This type of support system enhances the quality of our lives and our experiences—just like our home entertainment centers enhance our enjoyment of music and movies. This is extremely important for you today–and even more important for you tomorrow. Study after study has shown that strong social relationships are essential for a healthy mind and body, while also enhancing our life experience. They reduce some of the bad effects of stress, and help speed recovery from psychological and physical illness. They also support our desire for longevity. After all, nobody wants to make it to 100 alone. Relationships sustain us. The following are seven ways to bring companionship into your life:

1. Eat with a friend.
2. Go for a walk.

3. Go to the gym.
4. Go shopping.
5. Go to the movies.
6. Go on vacation.
7. Devote yourself to a cause.

The *Journal of the American Medical Association* recently reported on a study in which several hundred volunteers were exposed to a cold virus. The study showed that the volunteers with the most socially diverse networks were the most disease resistant—only 35 percent of the volunteers with six or more close relationships caught the cold. But 65 percent of the volunteers with three or fewer close relationships caught it. You may have also read the recent study showing the potent, positive effect that support groups have on breast cancer patients, improving their healing ability. It's exciting news to know that good support is not only more fun, but it also makes a difference. It's exciting to know that so many factors that affect our quality of life are under our control.

Now it is time to establish the support that you'll need for life. You may be pretty adept at this. Or you may be starting out—or going through a transition—and need some guidance. A support system is really pretty easy to create. However, it's going to require an investment of time.

The place you begin is with yourself. As I'm sure you've heard before, this is one of the most important relationships you'll ever have. The way you treat yourself is reflected in all of your key relationships. You magnetically attract people and circumstances into your life based on the energy and effort you put into nurturing them. If you ever happen to wake up one day and realize that you've ended up in the wrong relationship—or the right relationship gone wrong—and it is time to make a change, the place to start is with you.

We've all heard the expression "You teach people how to treat you." They watch how you treat yourself and learn from you how you like to be treated. If you are surrounded by people who are abusive to you, ask yourself, "Am I one of them?" One of the things you may notice is that if you have implemented the strategies on energy we have discussed, stopped destructive habits that were killing you, adopted the Health Care Hierarchy, and implemented a self-care and health care regimen, wrongs that others have committed against you will begin to stand out like a sore thumb. They will become more noticeable and intolerable to you, just like the person who finally quits smoking detests the smell of cigarette smoke.

Centenarian Secret   Understand that healthy relationships are adaptive. You should always be able to connect with the world, and the people in your world, in a way that is authentic. Expect that some of your relationships will change over time. Let it happen. Continue to add people to your life who support the healthiest side of you. Discern who has your best interests at heart and make yourself one of those people.

START BY SUPPORTING YOURSELF

Many people don't realize we have the power to attract into our lives exactly what we need. You attract what you need by nurturing yourself and staying true to yourself—by being authentic. Don't look for someone else to make it all better. Have patience. And most importantly, don't hide your true nature. Nurture it.

One of my clients runs her own business, is a single mom, and the breadwinner for her family. She was always trying to figure out how to handle everything and kept looking outside herself for support, but she was never able to find what she needed. She kept hoping that a knight in shining armor would save her. She felt that she needed outside support to get things under control and change her life. Several times she made comments to me such as, "I don't know how much longer I can go on like this."

One day, in a coaching session, I told her, "You're not going to get the support you need until you are willing to support yourself." I then asked her to consider this: "If you were the only place where support existed, what would you do differently today? How would you give yourself the support you need?"

She said, "I'd start my days differently by taking some time for myself early in the morning before the kids get up. When I take my son to baseball practice, I'd exercise instead of simply sitting there—waiting for practice to be over." She also said she would make a staff change because one of her employees was not working up to par, which was draining. This employee was actually creating more work and stress for her.

She said she would also create relationships that would support her in taking care of the kids' activities—including carpools and tutorials. She said she would take a vacation and go to a spa at least twice a year to really pamper herself. And she also said that she would spend more time thinking through the upcoming week so that her days would have order to them and would go more smoothly. At that time, she was kind of randomly attacking her days—with the hopes of surviving another one.

I was amazed by how easy it was for her to come up with so many ideas. She knew what she needed to do. But she was still frantically looking for answers outside of herself. I'm not sure why this happens, but you see this so often. Maybe this is because we live in a society that promises quick fixes for almost everything. So our first reaction in a time of crisis is to grasp for quick-fix solutions, which invariably will make things seem better temporarily while the underlying challenges persist. Instead of attracting the support you need, you end up repelling it. Sometimes the rock solid support arrives in a form that you weren't expecting and you end up rejecting it.

When you are under stress, your mind can become narrowly focused. As a result, you miss opportunities and solutions that are right in front of you. This is why it is so important to nurture yourself—especially during times of transition. When you focus on attracting solutions instead of scrambling to grasp for them, you are receptive to the good stuff that will invariably come your way naturally. Building on that is how you will ultimately transition to a better place and attract the support you are looking for.

Support Yourself Through Your Choices

Once you know how to support yourself—which for many of us takes the first 30, 40, or 50 years of our lives—it becomes easier to ask for the right type of support from others.

You may be the kind of person who needs quiet time. Ask for it. You may need to exercise in a way that's different from your partner. Go for it. Do the things that you need to do for yourself and you'll discover that you have so much more to give to your relationships.

▶ **LIVE LONG AND STRONG EXERCISE**

If you were the only person in your life where support existed, what would you change immediately to ensure that you get the support you need:

1. _____

_____

_____

2. _____

_____

_____

3. _____

_____

_____

4. _____

_____

_____

5. _____

_____

_____

Living the 100-Year Lifestyle Fay Litsky of Margate, Florida, advises: "You have to be healthy first. I've always taken care of myself. Nobody else will do it for me," says Fay, who turned 93 this year.

Be honest about who you are and what you want. Your willingness to let your voice be heard will give you the opportunity to make the rest of your life the best.

SUPPORT YOURSELF: ESTABLISH A PERSONAL RENEWAL RECIPE

Have you ever returned home from a vacation and felt completely refreshed? Have you ever said to someone you love, "I feel like a new person"? Well, what were you doing when that happened? What made you feel that way? *What if you set up your life with this renewal in mind?*

Wouldn't it be great if your work gave you a sense of renewal, fed your passion, and stimulated your mind as well as your pocketbook? Wouldn't it be exciting if the rest of your daily routines did the same? Making personal renewal a part of your lifestyle is what will surely keep your mind, body, and spirit young, regardless of your age.

Support and Renew Your Body Through Movement

A great first action when you wake up in the morning is to move every joint in your body. Stand up straight with your feet together and breathe in—as deep as you can. Hold it in for five seconds. Feel the air enter spaces in your lungs you don't normally utilize. As the air enters, raise your arms above your head. After five seconds, blow the air out hard while you lower your arms—again to the count of five.

Repeat this exercise five times with your eyes closed and then begin to move every part of your body—one at a time, beginning with the top of your head. Roll your eyes in a clockwise direction and then reverse. Do the same with your neck, slowly rolling it in a full range of motion and then reversing it. Do each direction three to five times. Scrunch up all your facial muscles by making a lot of funny faces and then release them.

This may seem silly, but most of us aren't utilizing our bodies to anywhere near their capabilities. This creates a state of imbalance and disharmony inside us. We are made to move through much greater ranges of motion than our twenty-first-century lives call for. When you start the day stretching this way, you will wake up your entire body and feel energized instantly.

Continue stretching your way throughout your body. Include your shoulders, elbows, wrists, fingers, chest, waist, upper and lower spine, hips, knees, feet, and toes. If you like the feeling you get from this type of full-body movement, yoga would be a fantastic exercise for you.

Every cell of your body will begin to wake up, and you'll like it. The cracks that you hear will remind you that you are not a kid. But assume your healthful workout is slowing down the aging process and just focus on working out the kinks. You might inform your doctor, massage therapist, or personal trainer about the places you feel the most kinked up so they can help you work through it and help you rebuild your body in the healthiest and best way.

Go through these motions two to three times a day and they will keep your body awake and regenerated. It only takes five minutes, but the awakening will help you feel alive.

I recently attended a car control clinic with my 15-year-old son Jacob after he received his learner's permit. One key point made by the instructor is that most driving is done without turning the wheel through its full range of motion. The average turn only takes the wheel through a half to one full revolution. This becomes a habit for most of us and especially for teenagers. Young drivers are actually often afraid to really turn the wheel all the way, which can sometimes cause them to experience unnecessary accidents.

When I heard this, I thought automatically of the way we treat our bodies. Our lives have grown so sedentary. We forget the multitude of tasks that our bodies are designed to do. A very important aspect of the 100-Year Lifestyle is to have confidence in your body so it can support you with any activity you choose. Making personal renewal a part of your lifestyle will give you the body confidence you need for the next 40 or 50 years.

While you may not be able to feel like you are 18 again, you'll be amazed at how youthful, active, and healthy you'll feel by making renewal a part of your life. If you ask anyone who feels old what makes them feel that way, they will often tell you that they can no longer do the things that they want to do—physically speaking. Their capabilities are less than they would like. You can get much of this youthful physical feeling back with full-body movement.

You also renew your body and mind through rest. Getting enough sleep, and getting quality sleep, is important. Have the right bed and pillow to support your spine and body type. If you share your bed with a life partner and you have different shapes, both of you should be able to customize your side of the mattress. You both deserve the right support for you. Also, if you sit a lot at work, get an ergonomic chair to support your back.

Take the self-care and health care strategies that work best for you and put them into your daily routine, and you will customized your Personal Renewal Recipe.

MAGNETICALLY ATTRACTING AN ABUNDANCE OF SUPPORT

The next level of support after the support of yourself is that of family and close friends. We often tend to take these relationships for granted. Just like the relationships with ourselves, we overlook their importance. However, you'll find that the quality of your life will skyrocket when you invest in the relationships that are closest to home.

Today, ask your partner, "What are the changes you are trying to make in your life? How can I support you?" Switch. Take turns. Really listen to your partner and then follow through to make those changes a part of your lifestyle. As a couple ask, "What are the changes we know we need to make? What action step can we undertake today to make those changes part of our new

100-Year Lifestyle?" Give each other the opportunity to voice what is important and then support each other in making the changes you know that you need to make.

Your primary relationship has a major impact on your health. Studies have documented the health and economic benefits of a happy marriage. And they have chronicled the cost of an unhappy marriage, divorce, and death. Studies have determined that divorce and widowhood create stress, which has been linked to chronic health problems. Couples or singles who live with aging parents or grandkids often showed negative consequences, in terms of their physical, cognitive, or emotional health, especially if their primary relationship is not strong. Keeping your primary relationship strong is essential to the quality of life you want and deserve.

The next level of Surround Sound Support is to connect with people who have interests that are similar to yours. Look for them while pursuing some of your favorite activities—like attending worship services, traveling, mentoring, spending time with friends, and working. Lean on them for support and offer them support as well.

A SURROUND SOUND SUPPORT SYSTEM FOR YOUR MIND, BODY, AND SPIRIT

A Surround Sound System of Support covers all of your bases. You should have people in your life who support you in pursuing the quality of life that you desire, in reaching your full potential, and in helping you through crises.

When you look at your current support system, you may find that you have support only for times of crisis. When this happens, you might find yourself on an emotional roller coaster. This should not be the primary way that you connect with people. Think of it this way: If your financial advisor specializes in debt relief, you will struggle to build wealth because you won't have the proper support in place. If you have a doctor who only treats disease, you won't have all the information you need to achieve optimum health over your extended life.

Surrounding yourself with the right type of support is very freeing for your soul, because you know you'll be able to make the best of every situation. Speak to these professionals about your goals. Discuss your long-term vision. Let them advise you, from their unique perspectives, on how to best reach your goals.

Multiple Circles and Generations of Relationships

One of the greatest fears and challenges of aging is loneliness and being alone. When we are younger and surrounded by children, their youthful energy can be contagious and make us feel young. There are a lot of birthdays to attend, anniversaries to celebrate, births, confirmations, bar mitzvahs, and many other opportunities to celebrate. Our calendars are filled with celebrations of the joys of being alive, with an occasional funeral thrown into the mix. This type of balance makes it easier to stay positive and motivated on a daily basis. These celebrations make life fun.

For many in our current generation of seniors and centenarians, they unfortunately experience more funerals than parties. When speaking to my 99-year-old grandfather recently about this, he was saddened about the recent passing of one of his pinochle friends. They would sit around and play cards together, for hours, on a regular basis.

The imbalance between celebrations and sadness can lead to depression and hopelessness for many seniors. Loss is going to be a reality of our extended life spans. The longer you live, the more loss you will experience. Unbalanced loss without celebrations to offset them can create numerous challenges, including feelings of loneliness or depression. If you only have one circle of friends, or one friend, you will put yourself in a position to be extremely depressed in the event of a significant loss. The more circles you have, and the more places in which you are meaningfully connected, the easier it is going to be for you to enjoy your longevity. You will be more able to cope with loss and stay passionately engaged in life.

We recently hosted a huge celebration in honor of my son Cory's thirteenth birthday. Papa Hy flew up from Florida to be with us, and when he got there, he looked every second of his 99 years. By the time he left the weekend, he looked 15 years younger, at least. Being around a different circle of people that included four generations of family, literally brought back his youthful energy.

Certainly, grief is a part of the process of loss, but when your life is multidimensional, it is easier to move forward. Building relationships with three, four, even five generations of people balances you and stimulates your youthfulness. When you maintain relationships across generations, you stay in touch with the radically changing world in which we live. This keeps your senses young and sharp. It keeps you active.

Centenarian Secret   Learn from the experience and wisdom of the mature and share the passion and zest for life of the young.

Further, don't overlook the value of purpose. Seniors who are retired and not involved in a profession, religious organization, or a volunteer group are at a higher risk of health problems, including depression. Staying involved in things that are important to you will give you a reason to get up every morning. Having several reasons to get up is even more important and much healthier than having a one-dimensional life without a lot of support. The more you give to multiple generations and multiple circles of people, the more support that will come back to you when you need it at times of loss.

Restructured Families

Treasure the relationships closest to you—even if they come in a form that you weren't expecting. Restructured families are becoming the norm. They tend to take shape with a lot of emotional baggage. You may have experienced this in your own life—or in the life of one of your children. Many people have a tendency to pull back from these types of relationships and resist the change intensely.

What would happen if, instead, you refrain from judging too much in these situations and reach out to your new family.

While I would not want you to compromise your loyalties, I would encourage you to develop bonds with children brought in by a new marriage, for example. It is going to become important for us to accept our extended families and develop relationships with their extended families. *Harmony within these relationships is essential and can eliminate a lot of unnecessary stress.*

These families are not going away. They are going to be a part of our lives for the rest of our lives. Accepting this and treating each other with mutual respect, love, support, and admiration is going to be important to ensure the quality of life we desire for 100 years and beyond. To resist this is a complete energy drain, like resisting gravity, as we saw earlier. Why bring the stress into our lives? Why waste the energy trying to control others or be self-righteous about our anger and disconnectedness?

Relationships with stepchildren and step-grandchildren can enhance the quality of your life and can assist you in developing a support system for your present and future. What you put out comes back to you. You can't expect to receive down the road if you don't give the support now. Understand that we can choose the amount of time we spend with these people and the level of involvement they have in our lives. But to deny their existence, and push those relationships away, just perpetuates separation and pain.

> **Centenarian Secret**   Our generation will be the first in history to have five generations in a family as the norm, beginning with the newborn baby, 25-year-old parents, 50-year-old grandparents, 75-year-old great-grandparents, and 100-year-old great-great-grandparents. If the <u>Discover</u> magazine researchers are correct, we may even see six generations with 125-year-old great-great-great-grandparents.

Multiple generations are going to have to learn to get along, work together, and support each other for the good of society as a whole. How can we do this? How do we balance our old-world values with the technological advances in this high-paced, rapidly changing world? To do so requires an understanding and appreciation of generations outside our own.

The other night we had our parents over for dinner. We were talking around the table about this very issue. I ended up, accidentally, hurting my father's feelings when I said that he was old-fashioned. But I meant it as a compliment. As I have grown into my mid-forties I have realized that old-fashioned values like prioritizing family, being spiritually grounded, and having a good work ethic, name, and reputation are very important to an individual's success in life, and to the foundation of our culture.

What is also important to him, however, is the adventurousness that comes from a youthful mind. Blending these values and accepting the gifts that each generation has to offer can build relationships that keep the older generations younger and energetic while keeping the younger generations wise beyond their years. For the older generations, they connect them to celebrations—from births to birthday parties to confirmations, graduations, and weddings.

My wife's grandfather—at age 99—looks forward to those special events with his great-grandchildren with so much pleasure. You can connect to these types of events through your family and extended family—as well as through churches and synagogues, professional groups, hobbies, and areas of activism with which you are affiliated. To benefit from these circles of generations you've got to be willing to show up and attend. Be there and participate with authentic and genuine goodwill.

Multiple circles might include professional, sports, religious, friendship, family, support groups, and others. I have seen people get consumed with one circle and neglect the others, causing an imbalance, boredom, and stress. Your Quality Time Living Model in the next chapter will help you achieve this balance and fit it all into your life effortlessly.

You may find from time to time that you tap some support systems dry. You veer away from the values shared by certain circles of friends. They no longer seem like viable components of your rock solid support system and you might consider letting them go. Disconnecting is always an option, but so is changing your expectations.

For example, if alcohol is a destructive pattern, you may need to disconnect from the bar scene. If you wish to settle down, you may start to disconnect from the singles' scene. Alternatively, if your family is not a rock solid support system, but you cannot disconnect from them, you may simply choose to reset your expectations with respect to them. If they are unable or unwilling to give you the support you need, stop looking for the support there.

Lifelong Learning and Multiple Careers

The first 40 to 50 years of your life you were building the skills to really maximize the last 40 or 50 years. If you are 50 years old today, think about what you knew and what you were learning 50 years ago. Think about it. Fifty years ago you were learning how to suckle milk from a bottle or your mother's bosom. Do you think you've learned a few things since then? Was your learning conscious? Did you choose your learning? During kindergarten through eighth grade, you embraced your environment and got to know how to interact with the other children. You also got to know some basic skills.

In high school you learned how to rebel, along with the skills to get you to college. Maybe you decided to learn a trade. Maybe you didn't learn much at all and just partied your brains out. Either way, you collected experiences that on some level have shaped your life today. In college you learned the skills to land a job or targeted a profession to work in so you could make a living. Now here you are with maybe 40, 50, or 60 years left. Do you think there are a few more things you might like to learn and master over these remaining decades? What would you love to learn? You have plenty of time to get excited about mastering new skills, taking adventures, traveling the world, experiencing different cultures, starting a new business.

Dan Sullivan, the founder and CEO of Strategic Coach, teaches that you set goals in areas of life that are of interest to you, and in the achievement of those goals, you learn about things that are meaningful to your life. Your goals actually become the foundation for your own personal school of life. What an inspiring way to look at lifelong learning. And if you are an entrepreneur who wants to get the most out of life, you should seriously consider his program.

One of my good friends and colleagues, Dr. Russ Pavkov, helped his mother Helen Pavkov publish her first book of poetry, *Through Sunshine and Shadow*, at 93 years of age. Helen worked with her grandson, Tim, to key her words into the computer and her daughter, Kathryn, did the book's illustrations. Her other daughters, Janet, Peg, and Carole, proofread her work and organized the poems into topics and chapters. What a great mutigenerational effort.

Embrace multiple generations of family, friends, and community. You will stay engaged in life and build Surround Sound Support to sustain you during your longevity.

When you feel the support it becomes easier to embrace the opportunities that the world has to offer, including new knowledge, skills, and adventures.

What do you want to learn over the next 10, 20, or 30 years? Do you want to master finances? Do you want to learn about real estate? Do you want to learn to ski, hike 14,000-foot mountains, or become an expert in organic gardening? Are you ready to see the world? It's your 100-Year Lifestyle and it's your choice. Let's get excited about a life of constant learning.

CHAPTER 15
EMBRACING YOUR PASSIONS THROUGH LIFELONG LEARNING

A new study shows that seniors engaged in artistic pursuits are actually improving their health. But don't pursue creativity simply to produce longevity. Understand that there will be seasons when you're constantly feeding your hunger for knowledge, feeding your creative drive, and cultivating your rock solid support system. You will also have seasons when you are growing your business, and raising your family. There may also be seasons when you relax and beach yourself. Maybe you are or have been in hibernation season, like a bear, and are ready to come out of your cave.

The important thing is to never hold yourself back from change because you think you are "too old." If there is one thing that I want you to pick up from this book it is that you are never too old to embrace your life. Expect new seasons to arrive somewhat unexpectedly. Take the time to think about all the things you would love to experience in your lifetime. You may be overtaken with a desire to do something out of the box. Seizing such moments is what the 100-Year Lifestyle is all about.

If Helen Pavkov can begin again in her nineties, then you can certainly begin again now. When chasing your dreams, think Change Principle Number 2: Progress, not perfection.

Change Principle Number 2 is so important, as the choice to stay in the game and not let the challenges get you down is crucial to reaching your desired goals. You never know which is going to be the final drop of knowledge and experience you need to make the most of your talents, passion, and abilities.

Letting go of past mistakes is very important for growth and progress. You must accept the challenges that come your way and develop a plan of action. An extreme example of this involved one of my clients. He began coaching with me after he was audited and ended up owing the IRS $200,000 in back taxes. It was simply paralyzing him. The government wanted its money paid back in the amount of $25,000 a quarter for the next two years. Unfortunately he was not producing the income necessary to meet these demands. The problem was not his business, however; the problem was in his mind. He was unable to see the lesson in this experience—how this was the lesson he needed to become financially independent. At first, he was unwilling to change his ways. At 48 years of age, he had not saved any money and he was smothered by this debt.

I instructed him to figure the $200,000 into his overhead, accept his fate, and go to work with a greater sense of purpose than ever before. I got him to see the lesson embedded in this experience. I told him to think of it this way: "If this experience teaches you to expand your business by this amount, after two years you'll have paid off the IRS and you will have an extra $25,000 a quarter to invest toward your future. That's $100,000 a year. By the time you are 60 years old you will have accumulated $1,000,000. Say thank you for the forced lesson, and change your life." As of this time, he is well on his way, and you can be too.

ARE YOU READY FOR YOUR NEXT BIG THING? MIX IT UP!

Are you hibernating? Or are you ready for your next big thing? What would get you excited about the next phase of your life? Choosing your next big thing will bring incredible passion back into your life. Expose yourself to new and exciting people, and bring the little kid inside of you back out again. Are you ready to come out of your cave and commit to your ideal 100-Year Lifestyle? If not now, when? Open your eyes. See the people who are there to support you. Once you commit to your next big thing, you will be amazed by how much support you will find.

No matter what your age is today, there is always a new "next big thing" to commit yourself to—what will it be for you today? A business? A charity? Travel? People you would like to meet? Make a list of the Big Things that you would like to accomplish or experience in your extended life. Meditate or pray over your list for a few weeks and see if you can gain clarity over what Your Next Big Thing is going to be. Commit to it and make it happen. Enjoy the journey along the way. The second you commit to it, your passion will surface and you will feel that youthful energy deep in your gut. You will attract the support you need to make it happen.

I remember my 99-year-old grandfather trying to figure out a VCR and how much he struggled with this simple task. For his generation, change occurred very slowly and technological change was not a cultural phenomenon. Embracing change as a part of your lifestyle eliminates the frustration that resisting change can create. Technology, for example, is here to stay and the one thing that we can be sure of is that there will constantly be new products, services, and ideas that transform the way we live our lives. We are fortunate to grow up in an age of innovation. Over the course of our 100-Year Lifestyle, we can be sure that this trend will continue. Continue to embrace them with a willingness to learn.

What would you like to learn over the next 30, 40, or 50 years of your life? Would you like to learn about wine and food? Would you like to learn about different cultures and visit them all? Would it be exciting for you to learn how to build and sell a company? Would you like to learn how to write a book? Maybe you would like to become a master of healthy relationships and learn how to surround yourself with them. There is no time like the present to begin making the changes that you know you need to make and to start setting exciting new goals.

KEEPING YOURSELF FRESH FOR 100 YEARS AND BEYOND

Make your life progress as one big thing after another and you will keep that freshness and passion flowing for as long as you live. Fresh energy keeps you young. Stress speeds aging. We have all felt the effects of stress on our bodies during challenging times, and we've all seen how stress causes people to look older. I remember seeing before-and-after pictures of President Clinton's term in office and thinking to myself how much older he looked. I remember the same was true for President Jimmy Carter and President George Bush. Studies on the science of "telomeres" may have begun to unravel the role of stress in our aging.

Making lifelong learning a part of your personality that keeps you fresh and minimizes the effects of stress on your body is important to minimize the effects of aging. Once you find an exercise regimen that works for your mind, body, and spirit, stick to it, but also read about and explore the latest advances in exercise information and technology. As your goals change, change up your routines to keep them fresh and in line with your vision. Don't get stuck in a rut of boredom. Change it up. Change is good.

Your Sixth Sense

Keep your senses stimulated. Science says we have five senses. Intuition is the sixth sense. When your five are sharp, your sixth is even sharper, and you will rely on this sixth sense your entire lifetime.

Centenarian Secret Keep your senses stimulated by spending time in nature. Notice every small detail, from the sounds of the wind and water to the colors on the leaves and flowers. Keep your senses sharp.

Throughout your day, connect with every activity that you do:

- Really smell your food.
- Feel the cool leather of the easy chair underneath your skin. Feel your chair wrap around your body and nurture your body through your sense of touch and feeling,
- Hear your environment. Really listen to the background noise in addition to the direct communication that is coming your way from the people in your life.

- Stimulate your emotion through music. Make music a more important part of your environment.
- Use fragrances to enhance your environment. Burn candles, potpourri, or cook with different spices.
- Feel your partner and let them feel you with both your sense of touch, and your heart. You will heighten your sense of feeling on every level when you truly connect this way. Sex is an exciting way to stimulate all your senses. How about that for an exciting 100 years!

When your five senses are fresh and on top of their game, your sixth sense will thrive. You will learn to trust your intuition, and you will follow your instincts toward your ideal 100-Year Lifestyle. At this stage in your life, your experience, combined with a heightening of your senses, will lead you down the right path. The top business leaders, athletes, and parents have all learned to trust their instincts. Keeping yourself fresh will heighten your senses and maximize the quality of your extended life.

CUSTOMIZE YOUR PERSONAL RENEWAL RECIPE FOR YOUR 100-YEAR LIFESTYLE

The purpose of your Personal Renewal Recipe is to help you stay fresh every day and make balance a part of your lifestyle. Balance is critical for your health and overall sense of wellness. When you venture out to tackle your next big thing, your Personal Renewal Recipe will be a healthy place to come home to and re-center yourself for your next go around.

When you achieve balance inside your body, you will find that reflected outside of yourself as well. You will make better decisions professionally and personally, your relationships will improve, you may even find your finances take an upswing. All of a sudden, once-dormant areas of your life start to flourish. You begin a hobby or sport that you have spoken about starting for years. Your efforts at work start to receive more recognition. You may even find yourself making a lot of home improvements to enhance your environment. So many of us give so much of ourselves and wonder when it is going to come back. Your Personal Renewal Recipe will provide you with a permanent energy-comes-back-to-you system that fills you up with the energy you want and need to continue to give to the world.

Likewise, look back at times in your life when you were under a lot of stress. Maybe you had a lot of work pressures going on or you were going through a relationship challenge. Despite your best efforts, can you see the ways that your general state of internal disequilibria filters into other areas? You may have made poor relationship decisions, or jumped from one lousy work situation to another. Rather than thriving, we downshift into survival mode when we are living out of balance. Resources feel scarce. You may find yourself being referred to as "selfish" or "self-centered" by others, and you may find yourself surrounded by a community of people desperate for things—grasping for love, money, or material possessions. This is a sign of your own internal state. Something in your life is stressing you and keeping you out of balance. Only you can determine the source and correct it. It may be a physical ailment, trouble in your marriage, financial problems, an untenable work situation, or even a housing situation that is no longer working for you.

Obviously you must do more than simply change your mind to change your life. You must make the changes. But the struggle is nevertheless an internal one that can be solved with your commitment to balance yourself with your Personal Renewal Recipe. This is a much better choice than the one to stay stuck and continue to go through life out of balance.

Can you see now why the most important relationship you will ever have, outside of your relationship with God, is with yourself? You will take yourself with you wherever you go.

While it is impossible to be perfectly balanced all the time, monitor your body and mind for balance, and make decisions to support that balance. You always want the pendulum to swing back to center. Your way back to "center" may include prayer or meditation, exercise, nutrition, meaningful work, family time, and personal time. Use the information you have learned so far to customize your plan. Your Personal Renewal Recipe will keep you in a state of balance to ensure the healthiest 100-Year Lifestyle you can achieve.

CUSTOMIZE YOUR PERSONAL RENEWAL RECIPE

Now it is time for you to design your ideal 100-Year Lifestyle Personal Renewal Recipe: your Personal Renewal Recipe to program your mind, body, and spirit. Every day, you want to strive for balance. When you live in balance, you will connect to the things that really matter to you and the world will find it harder to pull you off course.

Having a Personal Renewal Recipe that you can rely on will ensure that you start your day healthy, focused, and centered. It will reconnect you in the middle of the day to that same rock solid center, and help you finish your day there as well. The way that you start your day from this moment forward will determine the quality of your days and ultimately, the quality of your life. Let's take a look at a typical day in a 100-Year Lifestyle.

First Hour: Renewal

What is the first thought, action, or feeling that you have when you start your day? Think about your first thought this morning immediately upon opening your eyes. Did you say to yourself, "I'm glad my eyes open this morning because the alternative would not be good?" Or did you moan and groan?

A positive first thought, action, and feeling are important to get you on the right track. Ideal first thoughts might be, "I'm going to make today a great day." Another one might be, "I feel younger and healthier today." Another might be, "It feels good to be alive and I will embrace the day. I will create opportunities today where none exists. I will enjoy a relaxing time with my family today." Positive and happy thoughts have been shown to keep people feeling healthy and younger.

During that first hour, which you may find becomes your favorite part of the day, take the time to connect with your spiritual self through prayer, meditation, exercise, inspirational reading, stretching, or any other activity that gives you a feeling of renewal.

Midday Renewal

When I was in private practice in Atlanta, Georgia, my practice got very busy. My office hours were 9 A.M. to 1 P.M. and 3 P.M. to 6 P.M. My patients used to laugh at me and joke with me about my two-hour lunch breaks. They would ask me, "What on earth are you doing for those two hours?"

While I would use some of this time for prep work—writing reports, returning calls, and reading through some research—I would also generally take a power nap during this time. This was essential to maintaining my own sense of wellness. My patients would pick up on that, and it was essential for sustaining our good relationship. After all, my days were spent working with over 100 patients per day who were either sick and suffering, or wanting to take their health to the next level. They needed me to be at the top of my game. This afternoon siesta made all the difference in the world for me and for them.

Centenarian Secret   Finding two hours to nap might not be possible for you, but we can all find 20 minutes on most days. Take the time. Make the time. Shut off your cell phone and e-mail devices and reconnect with your center for your midday renewal.

In many parts of the world, siestas are part of the culture. Everything closes down for two hours midday. Our bodies are not designed to be constantly "on" throughout the day. Siestas allow people to remain fresh—in the mornings and in the afternoons. Also, sitting on your tail for ten hours a day strains your spine, muscles, nervous system, and adrenal glands—it causes a tremendous amount of stress. This can lead to burnout in a hurry. Taking the midday break, meditating, relaxing our minds and our bodies, can keep us at the top of our game.

When you get off track with your daily renewal, remember Change Principle Number 2 (Change happens one choice at a time—think progress, not perfection), and get back on track with your next choice.

Nighttime Renewal

This is a great time to spend time with family and friends, reading inspirational books and literature, reviewing your goals, reviewing the day, preparing for tomorrow, praying, or learning something new. Go to bed after you have tied up loose ends—this creates peace of mind and frees up your energy. Incomplete tasks can pile up and burden you through the night—lowering your energy and your capacity to embrace the opportunities and challenges of the day.

What would be the ideal way to end your days? Do you like to end your days with a workout, or by gathering with your friends or family? To ensure your ideal 100-Year lifestyle, it is important that you make choices for how you start and end your days.

Rock solid support comes from knowing how to support yourself, being willing to support others, and being involved with people. It is very important to invest your time in the people and relationships that are important to you. Lifelong learning can be a catalyst for steady growth and companionship. How do you balance it all with so much going on in your life? With Quality Time Living, of course, as you will see in the next chapter.

THE 100-YEAR LIFESTYLE
ACTION PLAN FOR LASTING CHANGE

1. *Support yourself.*
   Treat yourself the way you would want to be treated. Set an example for others. Apply the Three Life-Changing Principles to change the way you support yourself for an ideal 100 years.

2. *Commit to your Personal Renewal Recipe.*
   Once you know what works for you, make it a priority and a part of your lifestyle. Define your early-morning renewal, midday renewal, and nighttime renewal. Don't compromise.

3. *Exchange support.*

    Be willing to give the people you love and care about the kind of support that they need, even if it is different from the kind of support you like for yourself. And be willing to ask for the ideal support that you need from your life partner.

4. *Establish Surround Sound Support.*

    Expand your support system using the Health Care Hierarchy, multiple circles, and multiple generations. Build your awareness of the support system you desire and the people and resources that are already in you life. Plug the most important relationships into your Quality Time Calendar in the next chapter.

5. *Balance your support system.*

    If your current support system is great for crisis but empty for quality of life, joy, knowledge, and health, spend time building and nurturing support in these areas. Embrace multiple generations and multiple circles. Step outside your current box. Make the time for the support you deserve.

6. *Decide what you want to learn over the course of your 100-Year Lifestyle and take a first action step.*

    Buy a book, enroll in a class, or attend a seminar. Make an appointment with an expert. Choose a mentor. Create a long list, since you will have plenty of time to experience it all. Learning things you are passionate about will add passion to the rest of your life.

7. *Six sense your life.*

    Really begin to take notice and appreciate your surroundings with your vision, hearing, touch, taste, and smell, as well as your intuition. This will open you up to fresh ideas and ground you on the foundation upon which you wish to build your 100-Year Lifestyle.

PART 7

Quality Time Living: Making Every Moment Count

Whether you're working or whether you're playing, make it quality time.

CHAPTER 16
ACHIEVING THE ULTIMATE BALANCE OF TIME

Did you know that there are 525,600 minutes in a year? When I first did the math I was blown away. Then I did the math for ten years. Do you realize that over the past ten years you've spent 5,256,000 minutes? And over the past 20 years you've had over 10 million minutes.

The number becomes astronomical when you understand that you may live to be older than 100 years. If you reach your 100th birthday, you will have lived a grand total of 52,560,000 minutes. That's a lot of minutes. The question, of course, is "Are you making the best use of the time?"

The Quality Time Living principles for the 100-Year Lifestyle will help you take your life to the next level and maximize every tick of your clock. The purpose of this Quality Time Living system is to fall madly in love with your life. What you want is control over how you spend your minutes. When you master the ability to make the most of your time, you are going to be very excited about the opportunities that lie ahead of you during your extended life. You want to get to the place where you love your prime time because you love your work and you love what you do. You love prep time as well, because you love organizing yourself for great prime times and wonderful play times. And you love play time because you are having more fun than you ever thought possible.

A NEW PERSPECTIVE ON TIME AS YOU AGE
When you are young and you are starting out, you generally will not have as much control over how you spend your time—at

least you think you don't. For the most part, you will be working for other people. You may have a young family. There are many demands on your time that may not be of your own choosing. But as you mature, and you develop a little more financial stability and professional confidence, you'll need to rethink the way you approach time. Time is a tool and it's a resource. The good news is that there is more opportunity than ever to achieve the ultimate balance through the Quality Time Living strategies of the 100-Year Lifestyle.

There are many great opportunities in this new economy for people who are smart enough to see and capitalize on them. These days, the most financially successful people are not being paid by the hour, by the month, or even by the year. They are being paid for their talent and by the results they produce. In order to produce greater results for yourself, it will be helpful to change your strategy with respect to time. Time management is a very important component of the 100-Year Lifestyle.

There are examples everywhere of people who have not figured out how to capitalize on time. Recently, I was standing by my gate at the Las Vegas airport when a doctor approached me to discuss his practice. I had just finished up a seminar where he had heard me speak. He told me that he was seven years into his practice and he had become a workaholic. He was financially successful but was driving himself into the ground—physically, emotionally, and spiritually.

His time wasn't his, and therefore neither was his life. He said that if he didn't make some changes, his life would come to a crashing halt. He sighed and said to me with despair, "If this is all there is, I don't want it."

We see this horrible imbalance very often today with two-income families who never get to see each other. They are working all the time and are typically all work and no play. They talk about business morning, noon, and night. They lose themselves in the process. Work is not simply a part of their life—work is their life. In my family practice I would see parents come in with their kids at all different times—trying to figure out a way to balance their busy schedules. In the process, they miss out on the extended quality time that they deserve as a family.

Centenarian Secret Your minutes are your currency. They belong to you, and how you spend them will determine the quality of your life going forward. Every minute you spend represents a choice—whether you made it with full awareness or not. Take charge of your minutes.

Taking charge of how you spend your time ensures that you'll live a quality, purposeful life for the rest of your life. If you are ready to master time and capitalize on this wonderful opportunity, you can affirm your commitment by adding these words to your human potential pattern: "My minutes, my life."

Get Control over Your Schedule

When you are doing what you love and enjoying your life, you experience a sense of timelessness. One hundred years will fly right by; yet, you will be present for every minute of it. If you are doing work that you love, have good health, and have a life filled with solid and loving relationships, you are very close to being there. But you must still change your perception of time to maximize the impact of your minutes. Otherwise, your life can easily devolve into any of the negative patterns we discussed in Part Two—with negative consequences such as relationship challenges and ill health. With the concepts and vision in place, but without the structure to achieve the balance, even under the best of circumstances, you will not achieve the optimal 100-Year Lifestyle.

THE QUALITY TIME LIVING MODEL

To achieve the optimal 100-Year Lifestyle, start by dividing your life up into three different realms:

Prime time:

This is about production. It is the time you designate to produce results, utilize your skills, and apply talents to generate value in the greater world. This is all about working in your professional life or for your favorite cause, and it is a very important part of keeping you sharp, purposeful, and productive.

Prep time:
This is about organization and strategic planning. This is the time that you plan, organize, do research, and lay the groundwork for superb prime times and fabulous play times.

Play time:
This is the free time you spend reading, getting massages, playing golf, doing yoga, traveling, going on hikes with your family, and taking vacations.

I remember when I first opened my training company and began teaching this time model to doctors. They were blown away by how much more focused they were with their patients. They started to take more vacations, play time, and found that adding this balance to their lives improved their personal relationships and made their lives more fun.

The challenge for me was that our company grew so fast that I lost myself in the process and got off track with my own prime time, prep time, and play time. While I had mastered this time model in my practice, I had not yet figured out how to apply it to my new life. By disciplining myself to abide by my own prime, prep, and play time model, I was able to get back on track when I reconnected to "my life, my minutes."

When you run yourself ragged, just trying to keep up with the demands of your current job—and your present-day life—you are essentially treading water. Every day at work, you are learning new skills, sharpening existing skills, and gaining new perspective on how to do things better. Unfortunately many of us aren't taking the time to process the information and get ahead of the game. We are always playing catch up. It's like we're eating a meal and then frantically moving on to the next meal without taking time to digest. We meet demand after demand, just hoping that one day, things will magically get a little easier. When we see the signs of distress showing up in our lives, we often crash and say, "I need a vacation," and run that much faster until a crisis forces us to actually take one.

On a bigger scale, many of us do this until the age of 65, or whatever age we have in mind when we are going to retire. We go ballistic for 45 years of our working life and than come to a crashing halt in retirement. This "all or nothing' mentality and mindset can really burn us out, especially when our time is out of control. Quality Time Living will give you more control over your time than you have ever had before, and your choices will be driven by quality of life motivation.

How Successful People Regard Time

You break out of this pattern by learning to look at your time very strategically.

Many highly successful people already use the time model we are going to discuss, even if they don't use the names prime, prep, and play time. Let's take, for example, one of my clients— a hip-hop and R & B performer and five-time Grammy Award winner. I have seen him intermittently for many years as a chiropractic patient. When popular entertainers like him are on the road, which he often is, they often do a different gig in a different city every other night, sometimes every night. This can be a challenge.

They get through it by dividing up their time. When they are onstage performing before crowds, they are in prime time. When they are rehearsing, they are in prep time. And they incorporate downtime into their schedules as play time. In fact, I first met him at the beautiful spa Chateau Élan in Georgia while we were both relaxing on the couch, watching an NFL football game while waiting for a massage. We met while we were both enjoying our play time.

Entertainers, like him, make optimal use of their time— because they have to. They are peak performers and many people count on them. Most of us don't carry around quite this same level of responsibility. Nor do we have the benefit of people managing us and showing us how to make optimal use of our time. But knowledge is power and if you begin to value your talents and choose how you utilize your time with the same intention as these professionals, you will notice a giant step up in your quality of life on every level. Your prime times will quadruple in productivity, your play times will be much more fun and exciting, and you will stay organized through it all.

We've also heard stories of entertainers, athletes, and businesspeople who, because they don't understand the importance of this balance or don't have a structure to follow, are constantly in prime time and suddenly collapse—ending up in the hospital and suffering from stress and exhaustion. We see this with entrepreneurs who do the same. They go and go, without giving their minds, bodies, and spirits the chance to revitalize and renew. Balance is crucial for creativity, sustained energy, and peace of mind. It's necessary for longevity. It's necessary for ongoing business success and the personal fulfillment of sharing this success with the most important people in your life and the philanthropic causes that feed your soul. This Quality Time Living model will give you the structure to truly have it all.

Remember Change Principle Number 1: Change is easy. Thinking about change is hard. The reality of Quality Time Living is that you can rethink the way you look at the days, weeks, months, and years to reinvent your life and make the changes you know you need to make, without compromising your life. You can easily use this model to make your priorities *the* priority, even if you are currently locked into a "nine-to-five" job.

This is how you get off the treadmill and start building upon your time and experiences. One of my patients, Bruce Blythe, a very successful entrepreneur who owns the company Crisis Management International, understood this concept instinctively. He would travel and meet with companies to help them reach their goals, grow his business, and be productive. He would meet with his team when he was in town, and he would spend quality time at home or traveling the world with his family during play time.

Like my clients, and many other successful people, he knows how to use his time for optimal results.

DON'T BE A TWENTY-FIRST-CENTURY TASKMASTER

When we feel like we have an endless amount of time to complete a task, we manage the task in a way to fill the time. If we have a month, we take a month, even if the project would require just a handful of focused days. Rather than letting our most important goals and significant results determine how we fill our days, many of us have become twenty-first-century taskmasters who are busy, busy, busy all the time but never seem to be getting anything done. This may be human nature for some of us, but not for the truly high achievers who want to be as productive as possible while also enjoying the most incredible play time in their lives. Become a Quality Time Living person and take yourself to the next level.

If I gave you 100 days in a row to get everything done that you needed to get done to organize your life, complete tasks that were weighing on you, clean up the messes you have laying around, work on your goals, and strategic plan for the next three years, could you be much more organized? Do you think you would get ahead of the game? Would you be able to formulate an action plan for your ideal 100-Year Lifestyle? Of course you could. You would love it because with 100 days you could put all the pieces in place to make things happen for the most productive prime times you've ever had, and the dream play times you've always wanted to take. What if I gave you 300 days over the next three years, could you really, really set things up and get not just your current act together, but your second and third act as well? You wouldn't need that much time. You would be done so much quicker than you ever thought, because your time was focused.

The reality is that you would probably need only three quarters of this time, 75 days a year maximum, to set up your next three years exactly how you would like them to be. This is how you should think to make the best use of your prep time. Obviously the way our world is currently set up, you could not take these 75 days in a row, but you could scatter them throughout the year, designate them as prep time, and over the next year, two years, or three years make it happen. Are you starting to get the picture of how to use the Quality Time Living model? I've just given you those 75 prep time days a year, or whatever number you think you would need based on your current life and your future goals. Your job is to think about your life and goals and decide on the number that would work for you. It's your 100-Year Lifestyle to live.

How much prime time do you need to double, triple, or even quadruple your income or production? If you had 100 intensely focused prime time days this year, would that be a good start? Would it take 150 days? What do you think would happen if you took these 150 days in a row? You would probably fry yourself with this constant intensity and burn yourself out. Is it any wonder that you feel exhausted all the time now if you feel like you have been living in constant prime time over the last 25 years? Think about how much more productive you could be, how much more money you would make, or how much more you could contribute if you took ownership over your time and focused your energy this way. What an energy enhancer it is to take control over your life with this structure that makes Quality Time Living your constant motivation.

Play time is where it really gets fun. From this point forward, look at play time differently than you ever have before. You don't have to earn it, you don't have to be exhausted to take it, and you take as much of it as you can afford to take to enjoy the quality of life you deserve for 100 years and beyond. Can you imagine taking 365 play time days a year for the last 30 years of your life? This is complete retirement. The problem for many of today's retirees is that they get so out of balance with play time that it just isn't fun anymore. They get bored out of their mind without the balance of a productive purpose to keep them stimulated. How much play time would be enough to give you the balance you desire? What if you took 122 play time days a year and balanced it with the prime time and prep time to sustain you and keep you connected to your creative passions in the work world. If you truly enjoyed your vocation so that it also fed your soul while you continued to earn income, you would fill yourself up in all three aspects of Quality Time Living.

As your financial situation improves over time, you can balance your schedule with the number of prime time, prep time, and play time days to support your ideal 100-Year Lifestyle. Maybe you have had a great run and are financially independent but are tired of the 365 play time days a year and want to get back in the game. How many prime, prep, and play time days would get you engaged in your life again with the balance that would also keep your peace? What if you want to transition yourself to a new job or a new business? How many of each type of day would get you there? Step out of your Monday, Tuesday, Wednesday rut and begin to label your days, weeks, and months with this new model of time and watch how your results, contributions, and passions fill up your days. You will find yourself using this language and you will love it. Your friends and family members will love it too as you take them along for the ride. You will refine your quality of life as you age in years, rather than retiring into the grumpy old stage in which many of today's aging population have found themselves after being blindsided by their extended life.

We have become a nation of free agents. Our ability to continue to produce value throughout our 100-Year Lifestyle now lies in our creativity and experience—our ability to bring new ideas, thoughts, concepts, products, and results into the marketplace. In March 2006, *Fortune* magazine declared "innovation" as the "main competitive strength" in today's marketplace. This is why Quality Time Living is such a critical component of the 100-Year Lifestyle. This work-smart structure will help you adapt to this new paradigm.

PUTTING IT ALL TOGETHER

The way to manage your personal and professional lives in this new economy is to manage your schedule differently. Let's stop thinking we need to fit our life into our schedule and instead build our schedule around our life. Stop thinking that one more sacrifice is going to yield the job security that you crave. It is not. You need to learn to work smart. This means managing your career around your life while you enjoy the balance. This will give you the upper hand—at work and in life.

Unfortunately for many of us, we are plugged in all the time. This gives us great flexibility in how and where we do our jobs. However, if we don't manage our time, we end up "plugged in" and "on call" all the time. Wouldn't you love to "unplug yourself" every now and then?

If you are not building enough time to play into your life, try "slacking off" for a change, not by goofing off at work, but by scheduling some real quality play time. This is when great ideas are born and when we begin to build our lives from a place of awareness.

▶ CENTENARIAN SECRET

What happens when your life is out of balance? If you have too much prime time and not enough prep and play time . . . you are probably reaching your professional goals but you are exhausted, your health is suffering, and you may be having challenges in your most important relationships, which can lead to resentment, pressure from home, or even divorce.

If you have too much prep time and not enough prime and play time . . . you are one of the busiest people you know but you never seem to be getting ahead financially, or have time to really connect to the people in your life.

If you have too much play time and not enough prime and prep time . . . you are either bored out of your mind and turning into a vegetable brain, or you are increasing your debt every year because you are not generating enough money to afford all of your play.

Get back into balance with the Quality Time Living Model.

Whenever you find yourself overwhelmed and "stuck" going forward, I want you to stop trying to address the problem by simply tacking on more prime time into your already too-busy schedule. You will generally find the solution you are looking for in play time. Step away for a day, a long weekend, or a week. You will not only find your solution, but you will also find yourself along with the natural energy to enjoy your life.

Focusing Your Time

You will love what happens when you begin to prioritize the "play time" component of your schedule—and actually begin to build your schedule around it. Start to make your life as important, or more important, than your work. You can set up your life to have a blast. As the quality of your play time improves you will find yourself more focused than ever during your prime times and your prep times because you know you have terrific play time coming down the pike. This triune of time will help you create the balance to maximize every phase of your life.

Play time keeps life fun, exciting, and balanced. I'm going to give you examples in the next chapter that will demonstrate how successful people balance prime time, prep time, and play time. I first discovered this system when I was busy with my practice, trying to provide the optimum care to my patients, without compromising the quality of life with my family. I had lofty goals for my practice, but I also wanted to coach my kids in T-ball and soccer.

I found that thinking of the regular workweek as "just another Monday" and TGIF (thank God it's Friday) just didn't work to create the level of success and balance that I wanted. However, I did find that when I focused my time when I was with patients—the same way that a professional athlete, entertainer, or neurosurgeon focuses on his or her craft—my success with patients rose dramatically, along with my patient volume.

This was very exciting, but then I ran into problems when I kept this intensity all the time. It caused a lot of problems in my marriage and kept me from being present with my children. It was out of the need to find this balance for myself that I learned to follow this system. I then refined it as I began traveling and teaching other doctors and business leaders about this model.

I have consulted with over one thousand doctors who have also benefited from this time management system. Many physicians struggle mightily with this issue. For many of them, they start off incredibly imbalanced time-wise as young adults because of the rigor of their training. And once they are finished, they are left with the burden of building a practice during the very same years that many of them are starting families. I have seen many people watch their relationships falter under the burden of this stress. You don't have to experience these challenges anymore. Isn't it exciting to know you can take more time off and increase your production dramatically, both at the same time?

TIME MANAGEMENT AND THE 100-YEAR LIFESTYLE

How will knowing that you'll probably live longer than you ever imagined affect the way you view time? At first I thought it might cause people to procrastinate. I thought they'd say, "Why bother? I have plenty of time." But just the opposite has been true. In fact, I have found that one of the reasons people procrastinate is that they say to themselves, "Why bother? I won't have enough time to complete what I start." Or, "Why bother? I don't have the time to acquire new skills or enjoy the fruits of my labor."

Your awareness of extended living will motivate you to pursue your dreams, knowing you will have all the time you need to make the most of them. Procrastination can be a source of incredible suffering. I have seen numerous patients put off the inevitable care that they needed, only to require much more intensive work because they waited too long. To make matters worse, they are left with more residual damage in their bones, joints, and nerves.

I recently reviewed a spinal X-ray of a man in his fifties who finally decided to alleviate his chronic neck problem and take action on his health. I showed him his X-rays in two parts. We compared his healthy bones and joints with his damaged ones.

I asked him how old his healthy bones looked. He said they looked around 30 years old. When he looked at the bones in his neck, he sadly said to me, "Those bones look like they are 80 years old." Obviously all of his bones are the same age. However, each part of your body ages differently based on how it is aligned and balanced. Procrastination has drastic effects on your body.

Procrastination can also cause suffering when you know you're capable of accomplishing more with your talents. Knowing that you are not living up to your capabilities can be a real blow to your self-esteem.

Many of us have spent the first 30 or 40 years scattering energy all over the place because of our inability to focus our time. We don't target it. We try to be all things to all people, even as our confidence and self-esteem slide lower and lower, or our health starts to slip. After all, this is a game you simply can't win. Build a life of integrity by prioritizing and focusing your energy on the things that matter to you and set yourself up to win for the rest of your life by choosing the way you spend your minutes.

Time is your greatest commodity when building the ideal 100-Year Lifestyle that we have been working toward.

CHAPTER 17
PRIME TIME, PREP TIME, AND PLAY TIME IN ACTION

Let's look at this time model in greater depth and apply it to your life. The Quality Time Living model of the 100-Year Lifestyle will show you how to balance your life to optimize your financial, professional, and personal fulfillment. The first thing you need to do is to look at your weeks, months, and years as something greater than simply Sunday, Monday, Tuesday, Wednesday, Thursday, Friday, and Saturday. From now on, begin to think of these days as prime time, prep time, and play time.

As you understand and master this new way of looking at time, you'll discover some exciting things. You will get more done in less time than you thought possible. You'll find that your play time increases in quality. You will get the rest and rejuvenation that you need and the travel and adventure you want. You'll become more organized as you plant the seeds for the ultimate prime time and the ultimate play time.

If you have never looked at time this way before, you haven't really had ownership over your days, your weeks, your months, and your years. Haven't we all heard of entrepreneurs who neared burnout and then decided to step back and spend less time at work, and then they really struck it rich? The reason is because when you live in balance, your energy goes directly toward your creativity. When you are constantly exhausted and stressed, your energy goes toward survival—it goes toward managing the stress inside your body and pushing you through fatigue.

If you are self-employed, I really recommend that you allot days specifically for prime, prep, and play time. That is not to say they will be 100 percent devoted to one thing or another. You may spend 80 to 90 percent of your day in prime time on a prime time day, for example, and then 20 percent on prep time. But in general, you want to make it a complete prime time, result-oriented day. If you are working in a job in which you don't have as much control, try to set up your schedule so that your prime time matches your supervisor's or company's prime time.

PRIME TIME

Prime time days are about generating results, building relationships, or generating money—to use your talents and abilities in more effective ways to create value in the world. That value will generate the money to finance your 100-Year Lifestyle. But don't do things just for the money. Do things you love to do and formulate them into a business model that finances your 100-Year Lifestyle. As you generate money, decide in your prep time where to distribute it, so you can move your life in your desired direction. Also, the quality of your prep times will have a tremendous impact on the quality of your prime time and play time. So, let's break it down:

- *Teacher:* Let's say you are a teacher. Your prime time days are when you teach classes. Your prep days are organizing, grading tests, and creating lesson plans.
- *Writer:* If you are a writer, your prime time days are spent writing. Prep time is spent on research.
- *Salesperson:* For a salesperson, prime time is spent in front of customers and potential customers. Prep time is spent on getting ready to spend time with customers, and on organization, reviewing sales numbers, and setting goals.
- *CEO:* If you are a CEO, your prime time may be spent meeting with your board, shareholders, or key customers. Your prep time is spent on planning, delegating to staff, and constructing the future of your company.
- *Athlete:* If you are an athlete, your prime time is the day of the game. Prep time is spent practicing on the field or working out in the gym.

- *Manager:* If you are a manager, prime time is when you are meeting with your team to ensure their productivity. Prep time may be spent setting goals, organizing, or researching a new business system.
- *Entertainer:* If you are an entertainer, prime time is the time you spend on the stage or on the television or movie set. Your prep time is spent on rehearsals, makeup, and reading scripts.

In any of these examples, if you don't spend enough time on your prep times, the quality of your prime times will be reduced. If you are a musician and you didn't spend enough time on rehearsal, for example, you probably won't deliver a good performance. Prime time isn't only about execution, however. It is also the time when we nurture our talents. My wife, Lisa, for example, is an incredible photographer and artist. Over the years she cultivated a photographic eye and a passion for art, design, and technology. But for the longest time she wasn't sure where her journey would take her. All of a sudden things came together. Now, during her prime times she has an opportunity to do what she loves—making multimedia masterpieces. Her prime time is on the computer creating masterpieces. Her prep time is spent doing research. You can apply this model of time no matter what you do.

If you fully embrace this model of time, it will radically change your life. One of my clients in Australia recently said to me that after implementing Quality Time Living, he cut his hours from five and a half days a week to three and a half and he focused and improved the quality of the care he provides dramatically while increasing his practice by $360,000 a year. I told him in a joking manner that he should consider going to two days a week.

My yardman listened to some of the audio CDs that I made on this topic and quadrupled his business in two years. You can do the same, and you will have a blast in the process.

On the other hand, another one of my new clients came to see me awhile back. He was burned out. I asked him, "When was the last time you took a vacation?" He said, "It's been ten years." When I asked him how his wife felt about that, he told me he had just gone through a divorce. This is what happens when people spend too much time in prime time. This is a classic, "all work and no play" scenario. It's very draining and leads to fatigue, ill health, being overweight, and broken relationships. Stay in prime time for too long and eventually you can expect some sort of health or relationship crisis to come your way.

For the rest of your life, I would like you to make play time a priority in your lifestyle. You don't have to earn it, prove yourself, or put it off until next year. You deserve it, and play time will come first when you schedule it into your life. So many of us run ourselves into the ground and collapse at the finish line so we can get away for a weeklong vacation, and then go back to work and do it again. Finding the perfect balance of prime, prep, and play time is essential for ensuring a quality of life as you age. When you schedule your life this way, you choose your focus and build momentum.

PREP TIME

Prep days are about organization. They are about preparing for great prime times and great play times. The trick with prep time is that you may not see the results of your work right away because you are laying down the tracks. This is where the discipline comes in to work on your life and business, rather than just be caught up in it. For example, think of a beautiful garden in the middle of summer. When you look around, you see flowers in bloom—red, yellow, pink, and white blossoms. They are fragrant. A butterfly lands on a cluster of strawberries and spreads its wings. The garden is in full bloom, showing its magnificent beauty and producing a sense of abundance.

The days that you are sitting in the garden and enjoying it with your family are play time days. Planning the garden to begin with took place during prep time. Building the garden was the prime time activity. Utilize this triune of time properly and you truly find the balance you can enjoy for a lifetime.

Successful entrepreneurs and businesspeople are masters of prep time. They know that when they set things up the right way, the right things happen. For them, their prep times are spent on developing their business model, marketing, networking, doing interviews, setting goals, researching new technology, and participating in panel discussions. They work on building and nurturing relationships that support their primary businesses. It can take weeks, months, or even years, in some cases, to see the full fruit of their labors in prep time. But when they do the right things, for the right reasons, they can expect to eventually reap the right results. This is the magic of prep time.

> **Centenarian Secret**   Have you ever felt like your days were a hodgepodge of prime, prep, and play blended together? When this happens you will find that you get half as much done in twice the time with quadruple the stress. Quality Time Living is a much better option.

The risk of prep time is spending too much time on the "doing" without generating production. That is, "pulling the trigger" in prime time. Think about the real estate investor who looks and looks but never buys—or the doctoral candidate who works on his thesis for years but fails to present. Prep time, for some, becomes a way to avoid risk. This is what I call "Constantly Busy but Not Accomplishing Anything" syndrome. For example, I had a client who was very hard to get on the phone. He always seemed to be busy. In fact, he was one of the busiest guys I'd ever seen. Unfortunately for him, his practice wasn't getting him anywhere but in a state of exhaustion. He never seemed to be able to get over the hump. Eventually, you need to pull the trigger and do the things that generate results.

PLAY TIME

Play time is simply about enjoying your life. On a play time day, you are not busy trying to stay organized. You are doing whatever it is that makes you happy and rejuvenates you—reading a good book at home or on the beach, going for a walk in the woods, spending time with your life partner, traveling to exotic places, and celebrating life. When you look at your schedule for the next 12 months, what I would like you to do is to start blocking off your play time days first. This might seem counterintuitive to what you have always done. Play time first is a key component of the 100-Year Lifestyle. Play time days, however, aren't only for rest and relaxation.

You need play time to cultivate your creativity. Your creativity is ultimately the force behind the exciting and passionate 100-Year Lifestyle you want to enjoy. It will not only be what gets you ahead in this new era, but it will also help you choose new and exciting goals and adventures that you'd like to experience. I'm sure you know there are a million forces at work to ensure you don't take the time to nurture this creativity. The tendency, today, is to push and push—to keep working day and night and to stay plugged in. Scheduling play time first is about setting boundaries. It is also showing the world, and yourself, that you value your life and your family, and you do so by making them your first priority.

Centenarian Secret   Play time frees up your creativity, creates balance, and frees you from the grind and the intensity of prime time. Play time frees up your energy, relaxes you, balances out your system, and produces a condition of homeostasis—a condition of equilibrium—throughout your mind and body. It is often where your next big thing is born.

Many people report that the creativity comes out in play time, which is why you need to take it. What's interesting is that when many of us are in a rut, we try to work ourselves out of it and instead we just end up digging it deeper. The way to get out of a rut is to step away and take play time. Life is not just about work. You deserve to enjoy your life. Have fun and lots of it. In fact, since you are going to have more time than you originally thought you would, why not have more fun than you ever dreamed possible.

Schedule "play time" days around important birthdays, anniversaries, Valentine's Day, and other holidays, including Memorial Day and Labor Day. And then if you know you are going to take specific vacations, mark those off as well. The next step, after recording all of your key play time days, is to record your key prime time days.

When people retire or settle into play time too much, they risk falling into a complacency or comfort pattern. Once again, the key here is balance. When you are young and working, you may need to be reminded to include play time in your overall life planning. Maybe you have played too much in relation to how much prime time you have taken and you have no money. Your balance may need to shift back in the prime time direction. However, as you gain experience and financial independence, schedule enough prime time to fulfill your passions and commitments, and to reach your goals. But just know that all play and no work can lead to vegetable brain, negativity, and increasing debt or using up your assets. If you have no purpose and you are drifting, it can take its toll on your passion for life.

This is why complete retirement has become a problem for many retirees. I know a doctor who had been in practice for 60 years. In 60 years he had rarely missed a day at work and was almost never sick. As soon as he retired, he found that he had way too much time on his hands. He didn't pick up a hobby or cause to get behind, and he found it hard to engage in his life. He developed numerous health problems and became very stressed out. When he heard me speak about this topic he decided to go back into practice for two days a week. It was a great balance for him and, amazingly, his retirement ailments cleared up.

CREATING YOUR PERSONAL QUALITY TIME CALENDAR

When you plan to achieve balance, you are connecting to what is really important to you. When you are young in your career, you might work five days a week and a half day on Saturdays, leaving only Sundays for true play time days. If you took every Sunday off for a year, plus two weeks' vacation, then you would have had 52

Sundays plus 14 play time days, or 66 play time days that year. As time goes on and you get better at mastering production, you might take every weekend off, which is 104 play time days—plus two weeks of vacation—which totals 118 play time days for the year. When you achieve financial independence, you may choose 200 play time days with 75 prime time and 90 prep time days. It's your calendar, your life, and your goals. You get to choose.

Get yourself a yearlong calendar and three different color markers. Designate one for prime time, one for prep time, and one for play time. Start with play time, and mark play time days for the year. Include all holidays, plus important birthdays, anniversaries, and school breaks if you have kids or grandchildren.

Next, block in all of your key prime time days. This would include big shows or conferences that are key generators of income in your industry or a cause in which you are involved. Include speaking engagements or seminars you want to attend—which may fall on weekends. Once this is done, block out every other "leftover" weekend as play time.

Next, block out your full weeks of vacation. You might do this around school breaks—including the winter and spring holiday sessions, Presidents' Day weekend, and any other extended times when school is closed. You may choose to schedule them over Memorial and Labor Day weekends and Fourth of July.

As your children grow and begin their own families, you might choose to schedule one of your weeks to coincide with your children's and grandchildren's time off so you can enjoy this quality time with them. If you want to avoid the crowds, you may choose to avoid these holidays and go during the off-season.

Once your play time is blocked out, fill in your prep time and prime time throughout the weeks to support your ideal production and planning schedule. It may take you some time to develop the routine that supports your maximum production, efficiency, organization, health, and energy levels. You may find that taking a solid week of business travel works for your health, family, and energy. And then you might schedule the next several days as play time. Maybe you like one month on and one month off.

As you move along in your career, you might even do one year on and one year off. The beauty of this plan is that it is extremely flexible. You cultivate a schedule to match your talents, goals, and the vision you have for your life.

Your Quality Time Calendar and Your 100-Year Lifestyle

Your ratio of prime, prep, and play time days will vary as you grow in income, security, and age. When you are in your twenties and thirties, you may find a ratio of 200 prime time days, 100 prep time days, and 65 play time days works for you. When you are in your forties and fifties and more secure, you may choose 150 prime time days, 50 prep time days, and 165 play time days. There is no rule as to how many of each you choose and you can vary the schedule as your financial life improves and you reach different goals. It's your year, it's your life, and you get to choose your own Quality Time Calendar.

Plan your schedule the way you want. Build flexibility into your plan. When you plan out your life this way, you can build rhythm into your plan and gain momentum for your career and your play time. Connect your calendar to your Personal Renewal Recipe and master your energy. When things are random, you have probably found that you never seem to get things off the ground. You are easily derailed from your objectives.

After a few months you will get the hang of this planning strategy. You and your friends, family members, and coworkers will find yourselves using this new language and saying things like, "I'm in prime time tomorrow," or "today is a prep time day." Not only is it productive, but it will also help you understand each other and give the people in your life the support they need.

Your Next 30 Days

The important thing to understand, here, is that how you spend your time is one of the key things over which you have control—that will directly impact the quality of your 100-Year Lifestyle. These are your 52 million minutes; how are you going to choose to spend them? Now, I know that you are busy. I know that you are a responsible person, living an active life. I know that you are probably thinking right now of a hundred reasons why you can't change the way you view and manage time. I want you to now work on thinking of a hundred reasons why you can get really excited about your life. I want you to operate on the blind faith that if you take the leap into your ideal 100-Year Lifestyle, and start doing things for the right reasons, you will love your life because you love the way you spend your time.

Fear and doubt are key motivators that keep many of us stuck. I want to challenge you by suggesting that it isn't your demanding schedule that is keeping you stuck. It is the fear that you lack value in the world without that job. It is the fear that you don't have an identity, outside your family. That fear is keeping you in the doing—it is preventing you from shifting gears. It is preventing you from setting healthy boundaries. It is time to let go.

Again, think Change Principle Number 2: Think progress, not perfection. If planning the next year seems like too big of a leap right now, start with the next 30 days. Write down the most important play time and prime time goals that you have over the next month. If there are any fixed dates that you cannot change, enter them on the calendar accordingly. Decide how many prep time days you will need to be your best during those days and block them out. Fill in the rest of those 30 days to support your maximum prime time production and play time enjoyment.

Watch your energy, your professional production, and your personal fulfillment begin to soar. Get excited about the opportunities to have more fun than ever and generate more income than ever as you move to the next chapter and finance your incredible 100-Year Lifestyle.

THE 100-YEAR LIFESTYLE
ACTION PLAN FOR LASTING CHANGE

1. *Get a yearlong calendar that also has a month at a glance.*
   Decide on your most important prime time, prep time, and play time goals over the next 30 days. Fill in your play time

days first and label them "play time" using a colored pencil. Then, in another color, indicate your most important prime time days that are already prescheduled.

2. *Look at your goals.*
   Think through how many prime time days it will take you to reach your goals. Strategically color-code them on your calendar.

3. *Determine how many prep time days you will need.*
   Figure out how many days it will take you to organize yourself to make your prime times a record-setting experience and at the same time, make your play time more enjoyable than ever.

4. *Fill in the rest of your calendar.*
   Schedule prime time, prep time, and play time days that will support you in reaching your goals.

5. *Stay focused on each day.*
   Be true to each day's designated purpose, allowing for minor overlaps of activities since you are new to this system. Mastering this system is a process that takes time and you should remember the Three Life-Changing Principles throughout the process and keep your ideal 100-Year Lifestyle in mind.

6. *Set up your entire year following the same guidelines.*
   Build flexibility into your schedule and watch your productivity and passion soar as you achieve the ultimate balance.

7. *Protect your time.*
   Make your play times as fun and relaxing as possible, make your prime times as fun and productive as possible, and use your prep time to keep your life organized to maximize your play times and prime times. Have more fun than ever, making the most of your minutes.

PART 8

Financing Your 100-Year Lifestyle

Package your passion and attract money for a lifetime.

CHAPTER 18
YOU'RE GOING TO NEED MORE THAN YOU THOUGHT

The 100-Year Lifestyle is the greatest financial opportunity that we could ever imagine for us individually, and as a society. As you know, a key element of the 100-Year Lifestyle is taking care of your health, so you can optimize your quality of life and enjoy longevity. But because of that, you also have the opportunity as well to remain productive, well into your later years, generate more money than you ever dreamed of, and contribute more back to the world.

YOU'RE GOING TO NEED MORE THAN YOU THOUGHT FOR LONGER THAN YOU THOUGHT

So, what does remaining productive look like? Well, I know of a man, Jack Cashin, who owns a polo field in Georgia named Chukkar Farm and Polo Club. He hosts polo matches for large gatherings and also runs a horse camp, gives riding lessons, and rides himself daily—at 80 years of age. He also continues to play in polo matches himself. He is combining his love of horses with his love of the land, and he is continuing to generate money into his eighth decade of life. He is a prime example of someone living a 100-Year Lifestyle.

He has lead a fascinating life, comprised of myriad chapters—he bought an island in the Bahamas, ran for governor, founded and operated a chain of restaurants, and he has modeled for magazines and played polo with a prince. We are going to talk a lot in this chapter about the myriad "acts" that make up a life. This is a new phenomenon we are now seeing in response to the population's greater longevity, and a new economy. Surveys show that the majority of people over 60 intend to continue to generate money and value in the marketplace. They plan to continue working either full- or part-time, as consultants or by setting up their own companies. In some cases, they have logged many years at a corporation or in a single profession and are beginning their "Second Acts"—pursuing a career that may be more fulfilling and flexible. In other cases, they may have pursued a variety of paths throughout their lives and are now on their third, fourth, or fifth acts.

We are definitely living in exciting financial times. Shift your perspective from thinking that financing a terrific, 100-Year Lifestyle is going to be hard—that if you live to be 100, you may run out of money. Instead, get excited about the opportunities and all the possibilities that exist in the next phase of your financial life and embrace them. You have the time to pursue a multitude of passions, paths, and interests and live your dream life financially.

Retirement is quickly becoming an outdated concept. *The Merriam-Webster Dictionary* defines it as "to go away, retreat, or withdraw." It was a concept that was created for a world where the average life expectancy was 60 to 65 years. The plan was to work for a company for 30 to 40 years, retire, and then go away, retreat, or withdraw from society until you die just a few years later. Is this your plan for your extended life, knowing that you may have 35 years left? How many years of a purposeless life will it take to turn your mind into mush?

Using the Quality Time Living model and combining the balance of meaningful prime times and play times is a way to refine the second half of your life to make your extended years your best years ever. Instead of *retirement*, how about we think of the term *refinement*? This next phase of your life should be about refining and mastering your lifestyle. You should be able to move with ease between your play, prep, and prime times and define how you spend your time so you are having a blast, making a difference, and maximizing your talents and creativity. That is the ideal. Boomers who have been surveyed on their retirement views say they want a "flexible" work arrangement that allows them to work intensely for shorter periods of time, with maximum production and minimal effort, while enjoying life to the fullest with as much play time as possible. Again, this is the concept of quality prime times that we've been discussing throughout this chapter, and it will help you to finance an incredible 100-Year Lifestyle.

Centenarian Secret   This desire for a flexible work schedule is very common for today's retirees as more and more of them are going back to work. Some key reasons that retirees want to continue to work, aside from generating more money, include a desire to stay mentally active, a desire to stay physically active, and a desire to remain productive or useful.

RETHINKING "RETIREMENT"

With all the opportunities that exist, why live off of your portfolio as early as your mid-sixties? If you wait to claim Social Security until you are 70, 80, 90 years of age or older, you will get higher benefits than you would at 65 while continuing to have purpose and utilizing your talents to the fullest. That's just one benefit. But why not also use the passions and expertise that you have accumulated over the years to build and supplement your income, stimulate your mind, and give you purpose throughout your extended life? These are important options and choices that you'll want to consider as you question whether or not you really want to retire, especially when you have the realization that through Quality Time Living you can take as much play time as you want. Choosing to work is a world away from having to work. It is the difference between doing what you love and feeling trapped by your circumstances.

This is a key reason why saving and investing money, throughout your working life, is so important. Joseph Cowen, for example, ran a successful business with his wife, Marie, for 30 years. They had initially discovered clay on their property and, as a result, started Sheffield Pottery. Cowen spun the pots and his wife designed the pottery. They grew that company to become one of the largest suppliers of ceramic supplies and retail pottery in the East, and their youngest son, John, runs that business today.

In his early sixties, Cowen started to look for a way to retire from pottery, in part to care for his ailing spouse. He began to invest in real estate. He eventually turned real estate into his second career after he discovered that he has a tremendous knack for it. He learned from his father, Jack Cowen, who was a great real estate investor also. "When you buy, you sell" he would say in his beautiful Irish brogue—meaning that the gains are always in buying at the right price. For the last 23 years, he has run his own real estate business and at age 85, he has 15 rental houses and two apartment buildings, which he actively manages.

If you approach your 100-Year Lifestyle from this perspective, you can also enjoy and extend your prime earning years. You don't want to slave away at a job that you hate for 40 years in order to save for retirement. If you do, you can pretty much bank on your retirement being lousy too. This is not the balance we are looking for here. Don't work yourself so hard that you end up losing your health along the way. In my practice I saw so many patients who lost their health trying to accumulate wealth in the first 50 years of their life, only to spend their wealth to try and get their health back in their extended life. You will have to pay a heavy price to get it back once it is lost. Achieving the right balance is what the 100-Year Lifestyle is really all about.

Second, third, and even fourth acts are a critical component of keeping the passion flame burning and the balance of your 100-Year Lifestyle. Sometimes they are even more splendid than first acts. Many boomers are starting new businesses in advance of their retirements. Your prep time is the time to begin exploring your exciting, new ideas.

▶ LIVING THE 100-YEAR LIFESTYLE: ON MY FIRST 100 YEARS

by Joseph Angelo Enea

As of November 4, 2004, I am over 100 years old—that's a lot of presidents and macaroni! Someone asked me about 25 years ago, "Mr. Enea, what is the secret to your longevity?" I replied, "Buying certificates of deposit that mature in 20 years." On my 92nd birthday, my son had a surprise party for me. As a joke, in front of all the guests, he made out a birthday check for $10,000.00, but dated it November 4, 2004—my 100th birthday. Ever since then, I've reminded him to have the money ready. As a matter of fact, I had it framed and hung it in the living room of my house. Needless to say, when my son came to visit two days before the big event, November 2, 2004, the first thing I said was, "Did you bring the money?"

About ten years ago, I informed my son in a very serious tone, "Well son, I finally got the lots." He thought I meant cemetery lots. After a few seconds of more thought, he said, "Pop, you bought the two burial lots next to Grandma's and Grandpa's grave in Frankfort, New York." Flabbergasted, I replied, "What cemetery lots? No! I bought the two lots in back of our house that that bastard Tom Morreallo refused to sell me 20 years ago! I bought them from his son, who sold them to me for the price that his father refused to accept before he died." It pays to be patient.

Speaking of cemetery lots, I finally did get them in Frankfort. My son asked me, "Dad, how much did you pay for the lots?" "Cheap! I got them for nothing," I told him. He then asked, "How?" I said, "Well, since Uncle George Congilero is buried in Phoenix and Uncle Johnny in California, Aunt Gracie decided to give your mother and me the two lots that were reserved for them, next to Grandma and Grandpa Congilero."

"Even in death," my son said, "you've got an angel."

If you're wondering, dear reader, about that $10,000.00 check, here's what happened. At my 100th birthday party at Grimaldi's Restaurant in Utica, in front of all my relations, my son made good on that check. He paid me $10,000, in ten $1,000 bills. The only problem was that the bills were in Italian lire, worth about $8.98, total, in American money. What's the difference? American, Italian? Who cares? We all had a good laugh.

The Notion of "Financial Freedom" Instead of Retirement

As you have seen throughout this book, planning your life with an eye on the future will spare you much hardship. Robert Sullivan, a certified financial planner in Los Altos, California, says that views on retirement and retirement planning have changed greatly over the three decades he's been in the business. The focus now isn't on saving for retirement as much as it is on working toward financial independence.

"This allows us to orient the decision-making process toward a time in our lives when we will be free to make choices and be less encumbered by the imperative to pay the bills. Our goal is to start liberating ourselves from 'job and career' so we can enjoy life more now, perhaps even feel 'rich' right where we are, without living a life of drudgery that ends someday in retirement."

"My dad was a great example. He worked two jobs most of his life—one in corporate management, and he owned a small machine shop. After I graduated from college and started my career in 1978, he dutifully became one of my first clients. I diligently went about trying to ascertain my dad's retirement goals and he skillfully dodged me for many years. He was enjoying his work so much it didn't make a lot of sense to him to be so focused on retirement. But he liked the idea of financial independence—having choices, control over his life, and choosing how he spent his time. This means control of the calendar."

THE FINANCIAL GIFT OF YOUR EXTENDED LIFE

By this stage in your life, you are probably in one of three positions financially:

1. *You've hit the big time and reached your financial goals.*
   You have all the money you'll ever want or need. You have accumulated assets that will finance your future, and you are in superb financial condition. For you this book was more about health, relationships, how you spend your time, and your legacy. You are less concerned about re-evaluating your

asset allocation, estate, and financial legacy, as you already have a team in place to help you continue to meet your goals. You meet with them regularly to discuss your goals—for today and tomorrow.

2. *Second, you might be on your way toward reaching your goals.*
   You have a good income stream and have begun to accumulate assets while paying down your debts. Stay on your path. Look to use your skills and talents to create multiple income streams. Speak to your financial advisor, insurance agent, and estate planner, and re-evaluate your plan for your longevity. Discuss your plan with your life partner. If you haven't reached all your financial goals yet, don't worry! You have more time than you thought to get in excellent financial condition. It requires focus, discipline, and consistency. If your goal is to become a millionaire, which is not as much money as it used to be, you might want to place a "multi" in front of it, lay out the path, and enjoy the journey.

3. *Third, you might be in financial trouble.*
   If this is the case, you've got to make learning about money a priority. You are going to have plenty of time to master money, so you may as well begin to make managing it effectively a priority. Check your credit score and learn what it means. Meet with a financial planner and commit to a plan. You have got to change your relationship with money. Not changing will just perpetuate your financial suffering. Remember, change is easy; thinking about change is hard. There is only one thing worse than financial suffering, and that is suffering for 100 years.

CHANGING YOUR FINANCIAL FOCUS

When it comes to saving for the future, set benchmarks and make your financial freedom a primary focus. Do you have a plan that is current? Is it real and based on your present financial position? Or was it a plan that you put in place years ago that is in radical need of an update? Start saving now. Pay yourself first. Do it automatically. And never touch the money. Also, urge your kids and grandkids to start saving—today.

Many of today's teens and 20-somethings are already starting to save money in Roth IRAs—an exciting trend. This happened in direct response to the nation's concerns about Social Security. As opposed to sticking their heads in the sand, they are arguably savvier about money than any generation before. And the benefits are staggering. Say your child saves $4,000 a year in a Roth IRA between the ages of 14 and 18—that is $20,000 total. If he or she leaves that money alone for the next 50 years—adding nothing but also taking out nothing—that child will have over $1 million saved in 50 years. It's incredible, but true. The obstacle for most of us is that we take a short-term approach to money that is based on a 60-year lifestyle rather than a 100-Year Lifestyle. We can only see what we need today. Readjust your thinking and open your eyes to the fact that what is good for you in the long-term is also good for you today. Can you imagine going through your 30s, 40s, and 50s knowing that your independence is essentially already taken care of because of the minimal investing you did as a kid?

What's great about embracing your longevity is that even if you wait until you're in your 40s or 50s to start, you still have time to turn your financial life around and secure your future. If you start saving $500 per month at age 50 and do this every month until you are 75, at 7 percent interest you would accumulate $402,189.79, according to Beth Thames, a tax manager with Babush, Neiman, Kornman, and Johnson, LLP, in Atlanta. When you consider that at this point your kids are independent, your home is probably paid for, your expenses are less, and your Social Security benefits will be higher if you wait a few years longer to take them, this is a splendid little nest egg to be excited about. Don't procrastinate; work your plan and get excited about it. Your best is yet to come. You can still live your dream while enjoying the balance of Quality Time Living.

Roth IRA Growth (amounts rounded off)					
AGE	AMOUNT ADDED JAN. 1	VALUE ON DEC. 31 (7%)	VALUE ON DEC. 31 (8%)	VALUE ON DEC. 31 (9%)	VALUE ON DEC. 31 (10%)
50	4,000	4,280	4,320	4,360	4,400
51	4,000	8,860	8,986	9,112	9,240
52	4,000	13,760	14,024	14,293	14,564
53	4,000	19,003	19,466	19,939	20,420
54	4,000	24,613	25,344	26,093	26,862
55	4,000	30,616	31,691	32,802	33,949
56	4,000	37,039	38,547	40,114	41,744
57	4,000	43,912	45,950	48,084	50,318
58	4,000	51,266	53,946	56,772	59,750
59	4,000	59,134	62,582	66,241	70,125
60	4,000	67,554	71,909	76,563	81,537
61	4,000	76,563	81,981	87,814	94,091
62	4,000	86,202	92,860	100,077	107,900
63	4,000	96,516	104,608	113,444	123,090
64	4,000	107,552	117,297	128,014	139,799
65	4,000	119,361	131,001	143,895	158,179
66	4,000	131,996	145,801	161,205	178,397
67	4,000	145,516	161,785	180,074	200,636
68	4,000	159,982	179,048	200,640	225,100
69	4,000	175,461	197,692	223,058	252,010
70	4,000	192,023	217,827	247,493	281,611
71	4,000	209,745	239,573	274,128	314,172
72	4,000	228,707	263,059	303,159	349,989
73	4,000	248,996	288,424	334,804	389,388
74	4,000	270,706	315,818	369,296	423,727
75	4,000	293,935	345,403	406,893	480,400
76	4,000	318,791	377,355	447,873	532,840
77	4,000	345,386	411,864	492,541	590,524
78	4,000	373,843	449,133	541,230	653,976

Roth IRA Growth (amounts rounded off)					
AGE	AMOUNT ADDED JAN. 1	VALUE ON DEC. 31 (7%)	VALUE ON DEC. 31 (8%)	VALUE ON DEC. 31 (9%)	VALUE ON DEC. 31 (10%)
79	4,000	404,292	489,383	594,301	723,774
80	4,000	436,873	532,854	652,148	800,551
81	4,000	471,734	579,802	715,201	885,006
82	4,000	509,035	630,507	783,929	977,907
83	4,000	548,948	685,267	858,843	1,080,097
84	4,000	591,654	744,409	940,499	1,192,507
85	4,000	637,350	808,281	1,029,504	1,316,158
86	4,000	686,244	877,264	1,126,519	1,452,174
87	4,000	738,561	951,765	1,232,266	1,601,791
88	4,000	794,540	1,032,226	1,347,530	1,766,370
89	4,000	854,438	1,119,124	1,473,167	1,947,407
90	4,000	918,529	1,212,974	1,610,113	2,146,548
91	4,000	987,106	1,314,332	1,759,383	2,365,603
92	4,000	1,060,483	1,423,799	1,922,087	2,606,563
93	4,000	1,138,997	1,542,022	2,099,435	2,871,619
94	4,000	1,223,007	1,669,704	2,292,744	3,163,181
95	4,000	1,312,898	1,807,601	2,503,451	3,483,899
96	4,000	1,409,080	1,956,529	2,733,122	3,836,689
97	4,000	1,511,996	2,117,371	2,983,463	4,224,758
98	4,000	1,662,116	2,291,081	3,256,334	4,651,634
99	4,000	1,739,944	2,478,687	3,553,764	5,121,198
100	4,000	1,866,030	2,681,302	3,877,963	5,637,717

REFINING YOUR WAY THROUGH RETIREMENT

The good news is that a sizeable portfolio is not your only option for a happy retirement. You will probably end up generating revenue for many more years than you originally thought since you will be refining yourself rather than retiring. Many of the current generation of 50-, 60-, and 70-year-old workers look to retirement so they can stop being miserable in their unfulfilling jobs.

This is not the 100-Year Lifestyle. Do what you love with passion so you never get tired. Do what you love and you will attract lots of money. So regardless of your current position, you should still have plenty of time to reach your financial goals. Still, this is not an excuse to procrastinate. You must start saving aggressively today, if you haven't started already. Here are some guidelines and information from the U.S. Department of Labor on how to get started. Use this information to help you refine your next 50 years to make them even better than the first 50 years.

- Expect to need 70 percent of your preretirement income in your retirement.
- Understand that how you save is just as important as how much you save.
- Understand that the sooner you start saving, the more time your money will have to grow. Put time on your side. Make saving a high priority. Create a plan, stick to it, and set goals for yourself. Remember, it's never too early or too late to start saving. Start now, whatever your age!

CHAPTER 19
CAPITALIZING ON YOUR PAST TO CREATE CAPITAL FOR YOUR FUTURE

Your past has taught you a lot about money. What you learned about money in the past affects how you make, spend, and handle it today. So examine your beliefs and your results. Are your current financial beliefs and habits taking you toward your goals?

The truth is that most things in life come with a price tag. This includes the basics like shelter, water, food, heating, and cooling—everything. Take long-term planning into account with respect to your money and manage your funds wisely, or you will be caught up in a survival pattern. Think about how you have earned money up until now. Think about where you have spent money in the past. Many people get caught up in a "competitive" spending. They try to keep up with the Joneses—at home and at work. Have you ever engaged in a game of one-upmanship with coworkers, friends, or neighbors? What was it like when the job was over? Or when the Joneses moved away? Did you ever wish you had passed on the new car or the latest gadgetry and put more in savings? What would you do differently now?

Capitalize on your past to create capital for your future. I've certainly made mistakes in the past. But those mistakes made it possible for me to achieve greater financial success, just as your mistakes will for you. Experts agree that for many people the first million dollars you make is the hardest. Once you've learned what it is like to make that kind of money, you'll have an easier time of it going forward—even if you've suffered setbacks along the way, which by the way, most financially successful people have experienced. Stock market losses in the past several years forced many people back into the work force, unwillingly. However, this turned into a blessing for many.

DISCOVERING YOUR OWN SECOND ACT

Your next act can be the most exciting and financially rewarding of your life if you are willing to embrace it. If you are one of those talented individuals who has been coasting for a while, open yourself to your next big thing. Quite often these opportunities are just waiting to fall into your lap if you are willing to make the changes you know you need to make. Have you developed an expertise that has value in the marketplace? Is there an idea that you are passionate about pursuing? Have you created a product, service, or idea that you can package and sell? You can utilize your past experience to generate additional capital for your future and have more fun than ever during the process.

Centenarian Secret   Do you have a passion or a hobby that you can turn into income? When your work becomes playful, you get an extra bonus in both fun and profit. This is one place where you will generate money through your 100-Year Lifestyle.

Put yourself in position to win and be patient. Be excited about the progress you make, every step of the way. Also, be open to third acts.

For many people, these additional acts are rebirths. You get to start over with decades of experience. This is the opportunity of the 100-Year Lifestyle. The notion of working into your early to mid-sixties and then essentially going on vacation for the next 20, 30, or 40 years is actually a fairly new concept, historically speaking, and seems to be a passing one which is good for everyone, including employers. A sizeable percentage of today's work force is nearing retirement age and many employers are trying to stay attractive to this demographic. For the last five years, the AARP has published a list of the best companies to work for if you are over the age of 50. To make these calculations they look at recruiting practices, training, health benefits, and pension plans. They rated the companies by work force practices and policies that are beneficial to this age group. The opportunities for talented, experienced, motivated, results-oriented workers will continue to grow regardless of your age. If you are willing to contribute, truly contribute and not just look for a place to hang your hat and bide your time, you will write your own ticket.

Remember the 100-Year Lifestyle financial philosophy:

- There is an abundance of money in the world.
- Do what you love.
- Create value for others.
- Create value in the world.
- Package this value in a business.
- Tithe by contributing money to make a difference for others.
- The money will follow.

What a great way to generate more income as you grow financially free in your extended life.

CREATING YOUR 100-YEAR BALANCE SHEET AND INCOME STATEMENT

The more you save, the more freedom and choices you will have. At some stage in your life, you really want to be able to wake up and say, "I want to," rather than, "I have to"—the creativity that can come out of that is exciting. But here is the idea that I really want to get across: It is never too late to start! If you begin thinking this way now, you will attract more abundance right away, regardless of your current age.

This is not just about earning money. It is really about feeling useful and using your talents and abilities to make a difference. The money will be a bonus.

Look at your current personal balance sheet and use it as a tool to gauge where you are on the pathway to financing your 100-Year Lifestyle. What are your current assets? Where is your money allocated? What changes do you need to make to begin to allocate the assets on your balance sheet for your quality of life as you age? Your balance sheet represents a snapshot of your financial position and the income streams you will have for the future. What do you want yours to look like during the different stages of life as you age? Meet with your financial advisor and commit to the changes necessary to reach your goals.

- Are you saving enough to reach your goals?
- Do you want to move from higher to lower risk investments?
- Do you want to change the way you are allocating your assets?
- Do you have confidence in your plan?

I was talking to a doctor who had been running a very successful practice for over 30 years. He was feeling lost and scattered at this stage in his life. When I invited him to do this exercise, he realized that he had real estate investments that were not doing anything for him. He also had flat stocks and mutual funds, and he was funneling his extra income into areas that didn't matter to him anymore and that were underperforming.

He was still working a plan that he had set in place 20 years ago when his values were different and his goals were different. Back when he set those goals for his future, they were exactly what he wanted. Revisiting his goals based on the 100-Year Lifestyle, he realized that his current plan was no longer a plan for his future, but a plan for his past. Not only that, but the world has changed drastically over those 20 years.

When I invited him to revisit his goals and meet with his financial advisor to discuss how he could redistribute his assets to finance his current vision for his 100-Year Lifestyle, he began to get excited and inspired. He began to see that if he refocused his financial energy and personal energy toward his future, he could change things quickly. He sold his property for a nice profit and invested in the mountain retreat he had been wanting for a long time. He took the extra money that was left over and reallocated those assets to meet his current and future goals.

In another conversation with a different client, he told me that he was stressed about money. I couldn't understand it because this doctor had a tremendous income. I asked him to send me a copy of his balance sheet so I could see where he was allocating his money. After 11 years in practice he had a net worth of approximately $1,800,000. His problem was that he had only $35,000 in liquid assets. He was taking his money and putting it into land. This was going to be a great long-term investment for him; however, he was concerned about the stress that the lack of easy access to cash was causing. For him, it was a matter of finding a dollar amount that would make him feel secure, and reaching that goal before he bought any more land. His sigh of relief was huge. I suggested that he talk with his financial advisor and lay out a plan for his 100-Year Lifestyle that would give him the peace of mind he was looking for, and I recommend that you do the same.

Create a balance sheet and income statement that you want to work toward. What types of assets do you want to have—stocks, bonds, commercial real estate, a business, or residential real estate? Do you want to change the way your money works for you to help finance your extended life?

Live Long and Strong: 100-Year Balance Sheet

CURRENT BALANCE SHEET	DESIRED BALANCE SHEET IN 10 YEARS	DESIRED 100-YEAR BALANCE SHEET
Assets		
Cash and Checking		
Money Market		
Mutual Funds		
Real Estate		
Businesses		
Miscellaneous		
Liabilities		
Mortgage		
Credit Cards		
Leases		

Once you decide how you want your 100-Year Balance Sheet and Income Statement to look, you can customize your 100-Year Lifestyle to reach your goals. These statements will give you a path that is filled with passion and financial abundance.

Your financial health will help to remove the stress associated with your potential longevity and get you more excited than ever about your future. When you have confidence in your financial plan you will feel younger, more energetic, and even healthier than you did 20 years ago, especially if you have been following the principles of the 100-Year Lifestyle. Some people spend the first 50 years of their life destroying their health to accumulate wealth, and then they spend the second phase of their life spending their wealth to get their health back. This is the recipe for a 60- or 70-year lifestyle that you should avoid. There are myriad

▶ **LIVE LONG AND STRONG EXERCISE**
List the talents, skills, and experiences you have accumulated that have value in the marketplace that you would love to utilize to finance your 100-Year Lifestyle:

TALENT   VALUE

_____   _____

_____   _____

_____   _____

_____   _____

_____   _____

_____   _____

_____   _____

_____   _____

ways to finance and create a sensational century. Knowing that you have more time than you ever thought to reach your goals will enable you to achieve financial abundance and keep your health without compromising one for the other.

Obviously, the best situation is to start saving for your retirement early—when you are young. The benefits are phenomenal—the $20,000 that your kids save today can largely fund their retirements. Of course, we all know how life can get in the way. House down payments, children, layoffs, divorces, and deaths all disrupt the most thought-out plans. That's why it's important to rethink the idea of "retirement"—today. Use your prep time to think through business ideas that can finance your fun and exciting 100-Year Lifestyle. The ideal situation is one that gives you the freedom to pursue your interests and the money you need to make them happen. If you follow the Quality Time Living model, you can build so much play time into your life, while generating money doing what you love during prime time, that you won't feel the need to fully retire. Many people have turned to real estate in recent years to start generating passive income. Your investments can provide passive income as well. And many other ideas for generating passive income may come your way. Be open to the opportunities. Of course, there can be a lot of hard work and some risk involved in this, and I'm not in favor of one strategy or another. You've got to do your homework during your prep time and think through your plans thoroughly. I simply want to open your mind to the possibilities and help you identify some opportunities that you may not have been aware of up until now.

Financial software programs can help you visualize your life financially. Not only can you use them to pay your bills and balance your checkbook, but if you set them up properly, you can also use them to view your balance sheet and income with a click of a button. You can see how your financial life has changed from one year to the next, and you can also use them to paint a picture for the future. Always remember to set goals to finance your 100-Year Lifestyle and use Quality Time Living as a means to reach those goals. Your financial health will enable you to contribute to your family and the world and pave the way for a living legacy that you can enjoy while you are here, and not just after you are gone.

USING YOUR MONEY TO MAKE A DIFFERENCE

Giving back to society is important because it is the right thing to do and it gives your money a purpose. One of my mentors told me that the hole that you give through will determine the size of the hole you receive through. Giving of your time and money is also crucial to your ongoing financial abundance.

One way to give is to tithe, donating 10 percent of your income to your favorite causes. You can also stimulate creativity through giving. Ask yourself if there is a cause that you want to raise money for. Brainstorm what you can do with your passion and talents to create a business that generates residual income for your favorite charity, in combination with financing your ideal 100-Year Lifestyle. Mark Victor Hansen, another mentor of mine, has mastered this model and teaches it in his book *Cracking the Millionaire Code* and *One Minute Millionaire*. These are great reads from one of the most influential philanthropists of our time. The amount of money we can all raise when we combine our heartfelt passions, talents, and our extended lives can solve many of the problems in the world. Let's accept this challenge while we also live our dreams, both at the same time.

There are so many resources available to you to make financing your 100-Year Lifestyle more exciting and abundant than you've ever dreamed. Embrace this opportunity with passion as you get ready to live your legacy in the next chapter and truly impact the world.

THE 100-YEAR LIFESTYLE
ACTION PLAN FOR LASTING CHANGE

1. *Get excited about the financial opportunity of your 100-Year Lifestyle.* Look around you and begin to take notice of the resources and experiences you have accumulated and how you can capitalize on them to create capital for your future.

2. *Start saving now.*
   Stop wasting money now. If you have not yet implemented these basics, don't procrastinate another second.

3. *Fill in your 100-Year Balance Sheet based on how it looks today.*
   Decide how you want it to look in ten years and list the five immediate action steps that you know you need to take to reach your goals.

4. *Meet with your financial adviser, accountant, estate planner, and insurance agent.*
   Review your financial plan and income opportunities, and make the appropriate changes that will help you secure and finance your 100-Year Lifestyle.

5. *Prioritize your own self-care and health care and invest in them.*
   Having the money isn't nearly as much fun if you don't have the health to enjoy it.

6. *Check your credit score and credit report.*
   Take the appropriate action steps to clean up any errors.

7. *Be a giver.*
   Think about the purpose you would like to give your money so that a portion of your finances makes a difference in the world. Take an action step and make your next contribution today.

PART 9

Living Your Legacy for the Rest of Your Life

Imagine a world full of difference makers.

CHAPTER 20
WHY WAIT UNTIL YOU ARE GONE?

The generations before us regarded legacies as something they left behind. But thanks to the fact that we are living longer, we have the opportunity to create legacies while we are still alive. And not just for a few brief years—but for 20, 30, 40 years or more, you will be able to enjoy, shape, and mold your legacy for decades. This concept is important for you, and it is also important to our world as we grapple with the reality that people are living decades longer than expected.

In a way, you are already creating a legacy every day. How you work, play, and spend time with your family are part of your legacy. The commitment that you have to your community and to raising your children or grandchildren all shape your legacy. But there is another type of legacy—the kind you leave to generations of people that you will never know.

Dr. Ernie Landi from Chestnut Ridge, New York, is doing just that. Twenty-seven years ago, Dr. Landi had a 15-year-old patient walk into his office with excruciating back pain that radiated around to the front of his chest. With every breath, this husky, passionate football player would double over in agony. He had already been to the emergency room and been prescribed medication for the pain. The next day he had gone to an orthopedic surgeon and was prescribed some additional drugs.

Dr. Landi could sense the pain of this young man from both the injury and his desire to play and help his team win. After a thorough spinal examination, Dr. Landi explained the spinal injury he had sustained, adjusted the young athlete—me—who

Jim McKay

Jim McKay just turned 90 and is a senior partner at a Washington, DC, law firm. Back in the 1980s, he was appointed independent counsel and charged with investigating Ed Meese. However, for the past decade his work has largely been pro bono on behalf of veterans and child adoption cases. He is living his legacy.

"I was appointed independent counsel in February of 1987 to investigate Lyn Nofziger, who was a high-level advisor to President Reagan. In May of 1987, my investigation was expanded to include investigation of Edwin Meese III—the attorney general of the United States under President Reagan.

Since the mid-1990s, I have done almost exclusively pro bono work which has provided me with a great deal of personal satisfaction. I have represented a number of individuals seeking to adopt children. One case in particular was extremely meaningful. Our client (a single woman) became the foster parent of a 10-month-old girl. When the child was five years old, the birth mother sought to recover custody of her daughter. I had filed a petition for adoption with the court. The child had received wonderful, loving care from her foster parent. It would have been a terrible psychological blow to the child if she had been removed from her foster parent.

The judge granted our petition for adoption. I believed that I had done something, which, at least in effect, had saved the life of a young person. That was a very meaningful experience. I cannot now imagine not practicing law. At this stage of my career, I am under much less pressure, and work fewer hours than when I was engaged in extensive litigation.

For many years, I have also been heavily involved with the activities of a charitable foundation, which makes grants to organizations concerned with the health, education, and welfare of children. The results of that have been very gratifying."

felt immediate relief and went on to play that afternoon without any pain.

At the time, Dr. Landi had no idea who I would become. He was just doing his job, his passion, every day. He cared for me the same way he cared for every other person that came to see him. Because Dr. Landi was living his legacy every day to the best of his ability, people around the world have been touched by his message through me. Still passionately practicing after 34 years in Chestnut Ridge, New York, Dr. Landi is living the 100-Year Lifestyle, and through other doctors, including myself, he is making a difference for people all over the world.

I remember reading recently about Bernie Marcus, one of the Home Depot founders, who had a vision to build hardware stores the size of a football field. Thirty years later, after retiring from Home Depot as a very affluent man, he continues to build and live his legacy. Contributing millions of his own money, he fulfilled another dream by building the Georgia Aquarium in his hometown of Atlanta. His partner at Home Depot is also

▶ **LIVE LONG AND STRONG EXERCISE**

What issues in society are you passionate about that you would like to see changed? List them here:

_____

_____

_____

_____

_____

Go online and do research on organizations that are involved with solving these challenges. Research these organizations and get involved with the one that most closely connects with your purpose. Or, if the opportunity exists, start one.

continuing to live his legacy. Arthur Blank purchased the Atlanta Falcons and turned that team—traditionally a loser—into one of the most exciting teams in the league. We think that people like this are too "big" for us to relate to. Yet, Marcus and Blank were out of work when they were in their forties, prior to starting Home Depot. Today, they continue to find new ways to make exciting contributions to the world and build upon their living legacies.

Peter Drucker, who had already built an incredible living legacy during his 95 years, just completed a new book entitled *The Daily Drucker: 366 Days of Insight and Motivation for Getting the Right Things Done,* just before his recent passing. His numerous books have changed the way people do business worldwide. In a recent article in *USA Today*, Drucker said that at age 95 he was reinventing himself. "What needs to be done now?," he always asked himself. He would end up with a new action plan, which he would initiate after asking, "What are the priorities?" He lived his legacy as well as left his legacy to the world.

Why not create your legacy now so that you have the time to enjoy it?

You can move mountains if you just have these two things in your corner: passion and purpose. Find your passion and your purpose and great things will naturally start to come your way.

WHAT WOULD YOU LIKE TO SEE IN YOUR LIFETIME?

What are you deeply passionate about? Do you want to build a building for your church or synagogue? Do you want to be involved in preventing disease or poverty? Do you want to build a company, which favorably impacts the world? Do you want to travel the world with your family? Do you want to write, teach a class, learn a skill, create art, or write music? It's your legacy; what do you want it to be?

At this stage of the game, what do you have to lose? Speak your mind. Get involved. Be a little outrageous. Rather than dwelling on past successes or failures, choose the next phase of the game. Look back and reflect with gratitude and appreciation and remain purposeful, driven, and motivated by your next big thing.

LEADERSHIP AND THE 100-YEAR LIFESTYLE

How you live your legacy will be determined by your leadership abilities. There is a Leadership Ladder with four rungs that I believe must be developed for your living legacy to thrive. These are personal leadership, professional leadership, community leadership, and global leadership

As you climb the leadership ladder, the quality of your life and your legacy will improve dramatically and the impact that you have on the planet will be extraordinary.

Personal Leadership

Over the course of your 100 years, you're going to come in contact with thousands and thousands of people. By now, I'm

▶ **LIVING THE 100-YEAR LIFESTYLE:**
Bob Hope

Bob Hope, a former publicist for the Atlanta Braves, now runs his own PR firm in Atlanta, and began creating a legacy in his thirties:

"In my thirties, I pulled together a group of friends and we commissioned the statue of Hank Aaron that is now outside Turner Field. I did this simply to have something immortal from me for Hank.

In my forties, I got involved in the Women's Sports Foundation because of my two daughters. I have been involved for 13 years and am now on the board and executive committee. I was given the President's Award by founder Billie Jean King and am also an inductee into the U.S. Women's Sports Hall of Fame.

In my fifties, I started taking a group of friends—there were originally six of us—to rural Honduras to help the people there with education, health care, and commerce. Now over 40 people strong, the Wilderness Bob group hopes to have 50 members traveling with us next year."

sure you've learned that every one of these people has an opinion about what is the right thing for you. Everyone wants to tell you what you should be doing, what you should eat, and what is best for your life. At some point, you're going to have to decide to lead yourself. Personal leadership is about trusting yourself and directing yourself, throughout your life, so that you can fulfill your destiny and reach the potential you were created to achieve.

Choose your Dominant Energy Pattern to be about your human potential. Choose the attitudes that attract health, happiness, and success for a lifetime; create your personal Renewal Recipe and follow it; and discipline yourself to follow through on what you know is right for you. Lead yourself with Quality Time Living, finance your 100-Year Lifestyle, and embrace

▶ **LIVING THE 100-YEAR LIFESTYLE:**
Dr. Mary MacDonald

Dr. Mary MacDonald, now in her sixties, retired from academia in the 1990s and moved to Georgia from Connecticut. She loved warm winters but missed the diverse cultural events in her native New England. In 2000, she and three friends created the Colorful Arts Society, Inc., to spur growth of multicultural arts on an ongoing basis in metro Atlanta and the surrounding areas.

In addition to organizing a monthly calendar of events—ranging from fine arts to literature to the performing arts—they now have a membership list that is nearly 100 strong. They have given scholarships to students with emerging artistic talent; partnered with a bookstore to do a benefit poetry night; won a grant to sponsor a drama camp for children; and organized their annual benefit gala with an attendance topping 300. She says that she was passionate about the arts anyway, so creating a nonprofit didn't feel like work. Her advice:

» Ask for help from everyone you know—from your lawyer, your accountant, your friends, and your family.
» Partner with for-profit organizations whose resources can be invaluable.
» Don't do it alone. "The world is your partner."

the Health Care Hierarchy for the quality of life you desire and deserve. Embrace the personal leadership that is necessary for you to reach your goals and use your talents and abilities to the fullest. Nobody can truly lead you except *you*.

Professional Leadership

As you build your personal leadership skills and test them out in the world, you'll probably have the opportunity to develop professional leadership. This comes with experience and is achieved by creating results. But how will you know if you are on the right track? How will you know if people respect you? How will you know if you are effective? It's simple. Look behind you and ask: "Who is following me?"

Do you remember the childhood game Follow the Leader? The leader would perform an action, and everyone else would follow accordingly. In life, you can gauge your ability to lead by looking back to see who is following you. You may turn around and see that nobody is following you. This is a wakeup call. Personal leadership is about embracing the characteristics that make people want to follow you.

You may look behind you and see destructive people following you. Do you have a group of alcoholics who follow you to a bar every night? Are you leading people to a new credit card with the latest point system, while you go further and further into the hole? This is a great way to learn your level of leadership.

On the other hand, you may look behind you and find that other leaders are now following you. Congratulations. You're on your way. This is a very concrete indicator that you have become effective at what you do. As we discussed throughout this book, have patience and expect some time for trial and error. Rome wasn't built in a day. Your life and legacy won't be either. This goes back to the Titration Principle we spoke about earlier. The notion of a 100-Year Lifestyle should give you a new, fresh, and exciting take on leadership. You have time to raise a family, earn a living, and focus on issues in your world that you care about. The better you get at managing the things that you love, the

LIVING THE 100-YEAR LIFESTYLE:

Helen Graham

Helen Graham, who is in her late sixties, is a practicing full-time psycho-therapist in Atlanta. She has spent her life building a lasting legacy in many cases, by finding ways to be of service within her own community. This is her story.

"I was born in 1939 and remember the air raids of World War II. I made rounds with my physician-father and wanted to be a doctor but was lovingly told, 'Girls can't be doctors and we don't treat nurses right, so don't be one of those, either.' So, I married my high school sweetheart who was going to medical school.

In 1974 a dear friend of mine died at the age of 33, leaving her four children to me as their guardian. This forever changed my attitude regarding dying and death and, subsequently, the privilege of aging. Her four children joined our family of two children—all six children were between the ages of 7 and 11. They are fully grown, well-adjusted, and good citizens of the world.

At the age of 30, I began participating in workshops about connecting with one's inner self. I also learned about ecological and planetary concerns, service to others, expanding worldviews. I began to speak up and devote time to causes I knew needed support. For instance, I began a drive for recycling in our neighborhood. In my forties—after a very painful divorce—I was a single mom to six teens. I met a man who embodied the qualities I wanted in a life partner. I married in 1985 and he was supportive of my going back to college. I graduated at age 45 and went to grad school at age 48, earning my MSW at age 50.

Now that I'm 68, I love being a mentor to others. I definitely believe in inter-generational living, supporting the premise: 'The way to time travel is to have friends of all ages.' I don't think I'll ever fully retire, though I may cut back. I love to play, dance, learn, and travel off the beaten path. I enjoy leading workshops on such topics as Living Vibrantly in the Second Half of Life.

We are all 'libraries of information and wisdom,' and if we die without sharing our life knowledge, that wisdom goes with us."

more good things you will attract. Before you know it, you will become a leader in your professional life, which comes with an exciting array of benefits for you to enjoy over your lifetime.

Community Leadership

Community leadership has to do with making a difference in your immediate world. This may be your neighborhood, a church, synagogue, athletic community, cultural community, or a community that is connected to one of your hobbies. Assuming a leadership role in the community will keep you growing, connected, involved, and inspired over the course of your 100 years. Community leadership will give you a sense of purpose and connect you to the greater good. Use your skills in the community to make a difference.

Every organization is looking for people who care about their cause and who are willing to get involved. Pick a cause you are passionate about and be a difference maker by offering your time and talents. The people you read about in the newspapers and see on television who seem to be extraordinary people are usually just ordinary people who decided to step up to the plate.

The opportunities are everywhere.

Global Leadership

Global leadership is about changing the world. By climbing the Leadership Ladder yourself, and then spreading the word to everyone you know, one titration drop at a time, this crazy world will change. Isn't that exciting?

What would happen if we all embraced the 100-Year Lifestyle and the reality of our extended life span and used our unique and cumulative talents in this way? This commitment to leadership on a personal, professional, and community level would absolutely change the world. When I think about how extended life spans are going to affect my children, my grandchildren, and my great-grandchildren, I think about the kind of world that they will inherit from us. And sometimes I worry. I don't ever want them

LIVE LONG AND STRONG EXERCISE
It's time for you to climb the Leadership Ladder. Under each rung of the ladder below, list three actions or characteristics you can implement immediately that would make you more passionate about your life and that would make you more of the kind of person that other people want to follow.

Personal leadership:

_____

_____

_____

_____

Professional leadership:

_____

_____

_____

_____

Community leadership:

_____

_____

_____

_____

Global leadership:

_____

_____

_____

_____

to be afraid to go to school because of violence. I don't want them to fear being attacked there, or anywhere else for that matter. I don't ever want them to find themselves in situations where they may be tempted to try dangerous drugs. I worry about whether they will be impacted by intolerance, hatred, and bigotry. And I worry about a "world divided," which will only produce terror and isolationism.

By choosing a cause that you are passionate about and working to make a difference, you will be changing the globe by impacting your piece of it. What's so great is that we have an opportunity to use our extended lives to make the world a much better place. Knowing that we have more time on the planet than we ever thought we would, we might actually be able to solve some important problems. Think globally and act locally for a lifetime, and you will be exercising global leadership.

MAINTAINING LASTING PURPOSE, DRIVE, AND MOTIVATION

Compare the stories you have read in this book to the one about Max, the man I introduced you to early on. Do you remember Max? He was the elderly gentleman who died all alone. Max was 100 years old when he died, and I don't know why he was so crippled, broke, or so alone in the world. Maybe he was predisposed to holding people at arm's length. Maybe he valued the wrong things in life. Maybe he experienced some losses in his life from which he was never able to recover. But my thoughts about Max inspired me to write this book. Max was a very sweet man and his life touched me.

I want you to enjoy an incredible quality of life for your entire life. This means making conscious choices every day—from now to 100.

If you:

Are working all the time and sacrificing your important relationships, stop.

Are financially just living for today and aren't saving for your future, stop.

Aren't taking care of your body, stop.

Think you'll never find love again following a painful divorce or premature death of your partner, stop.

Think you are done contributing to the world by the time you reach "retirement," stop.

Are busy trying to control other people or are allowing others to control you, stop.

Are angry about the past, stop.

Are playing the victim, stop.

You deserve to have it all and experience life to the fullest, and you will have plenty of time to make it happen. Although it might be a little scary starting over at your stage of life, start over anyway and cultivate courage and energy-enhancing attitudes that become a way of life and part of your new 100-Year human potential pattern.

When you focus your life on things that are meaningful to you, you will have a lasting drive. Being passionate about your life is the key to mastering your life. Commit to things greater than yourself. You'll discover that messy details in your life start to right themselves on their own. You'll find answers. Ruminating is the surest way to stay stuck. Recently, *USA Today Weekend* reported that a Dutch psychologist tried to figure out what separated chess masters from chess grand masters. He subjected groups of each to a battery of tests, including IQ, memory, and spatial reasoning. He found no testing difference between them. The only difference was that grand masters simply loved chess more. They had more passion and commitment to the game of chess.

To understand the value of passion, just look at many married couples. I have a friend whose grandparents died within nine months of each other. He was 93 and she was 88. What was remarkable was that her grandmother had cardiovascular disease.

Her health was deteriorating year by year, but her greatest concern was staying alive for her husband. He lacked her gregariousness and she worried about him being lonely. When he began to succumb to poor health, so did she. She ended up living through his passing and spent one more Christmas with her family. The sniffles she developed just prior to that holiday became pneumonia by January. She was ready to let go. And she did. But her physicians agree that it was largely her willpower that allowed her to live that long. She had a purpose.

Your purpose is your choice. There are so many ways you can make a difference in the world with your unique talents and abilities. The world is waiting for you to step up to the plate. Start climbing that ladder and enjoy the view from the top.

CHAPTER 21
FROM GENERATION TO GENERATION—
FOR 100 YEARS AND BEYOND

When my children were in grade school they had to do a family tree project. I remember teaching them a little about my grandparents. But in reality, I hardly knew them. They passed away when I was relatively young. My kids also asked me about my great-grandparents. I knew a few details about them, but not too much. A few facts had been passed down. But otherwise, my mind was pretty much a blank slate. I basically knew nothing about them. They lived for decades and I'm sure shared many of my same joys and struggles. My kids' lesson made me wonder at the time about their lives. What were they like? What motivated them? What were their likes and dislikes? It would have been great to get to know them better.

Our longevity may be blessed with the opportunity to know many future generations of our family. I remember watching my Papa Hy get on the floor and play passionately with his great-grandchildren when they were small. This was about ten years ago. He is turning 100 this year, but their youthful exuberance still makes him feel young. In fact, he feeds off of it. He gives it back to them through his playfulness. The energy exchange was intense for everyone. He is very lucky to be blessed with the health to be able to do this. At nearly 100 he is still active and attends a weekly card game. He is getting to 100 with no knowledge or thought that he would live this long. He got here by accident.

We are getting the advance notice that our parents and grand-parents never received that we will probably live longer than we ever thought that we would. What will you do with this information? You and I have the opportunity to get there with purpose. Let's make our time really matter.

Centenarian Secret   We all have a history. I don't want yours and you don't want mine. What's more important than your history is your commitment.

ANTIAGING AND ACTIVISM

Get involved and select your cause. Whether it's working for your church or synagogue, the environment, children, women's rights, poverty, homelessness, AIDS prevention—pick something that matters to you and get involved. Make a difference in your own little piece of the world. Find a few causes close to home and start making an impact. Don't assume your voice is of no consequence. Don't curse the direction in which the world is moving. Put your paddle in the water and start rowing.

Your voice absolutely does matter. Several years ago I was flying back from speaking at a seminar. My neighbor on the plane was a woman who was feeling suppressed in her marriage and did not feel free to express her voice in her marriage, or anywhere else for that matter. As she tried to talk about it, her voice kept getting weaker, as if her throat were closing up. I asked her to shift her posture to a confident position while she wiped the negativity from her throat by gently and artistically waving her fingers across her Adam's apple, and then tossing the pain aside. She did it. Instantly her voice got stronger. I suggested that she sit or stand confidently and repeat this motion each time she wants to express herself and she feels her voice locking up. She followed my suggestion and today she is working in a new job selling a computer software program, and through her job she has to give one-hour sales presentations to potential customers. She found her voice all right, and you should find yours.

You will love finding your voice and when you do, it will change your life forever. One of my clients recently attended a two-day "Master Your Speaking Skills—Intensive" seminar that I give twice a year. I teach professionals how to master communication and public speaking. This woman was so terrified of expressing herself that she was in the bathroom crying during part of the seminar, terrified to take her turn on the platform. She eventually took her turn, though, and had a huge breakthrough. Now she embraces the opportunity to lead training sessions for doctors and has taken a much more active role as a leader in her community. All because she found her voice and decided to use it. You should as well.

Respect the generational shifts. Learn about societal changes and why they are taking place. Be a good listener and learn as much as you can while you also respect your own experiences. Know that you bring something unique to the table. Find a way to be heard. Now, I understand that sometimes the world can look or feel like an awfully big place. We can feel powerless. But by getting involved in the causes that matter to you, the world will feel much more like an extended community. You will become part of something bigger. You will experience the joy of making a positive contribution in your corner of the world. An important part of aging well is to always keep a sense of purpose. Always.

Involvement makes your life matter, brings joy versus complacency, and keeps it fun.

You can stay with the same cause for months, years, and decades, or you can rotate your time and energy on a project basis—the choice is up to you. The important thing is that you get involved in something bigger than yourself. You will meet new people, make new friends, and create new business opportunities. But more than anything, you will bring new meaning to your life. Just be sure to pick causes that really resonate with your soul. Don't simply join a group or volunteer for a blood drive and expect your life to change overnight! In fact, identifying causes that are meaningful to you can take a little soul-searching. The key is to get involved.

Mary Lou Ciulla

Mary Lou Ciulla, 63, lost her husband, Frank, in a terrorist attack on December 21, 1988. He was a passenger on Pan Am flight 103, which exploded over Lockerbie, Scotland.

"I experienced a myriad of emotions the day I found out my husband died. Emotionally, I was just in shock. There was no anger, initially. There was, however, a tremendous longing to have been with him. I felt profound sadness that he was alone that day—so far from home and in the company of strangers—when he was murdered. He was a brilliant, kind, and compassionate man. And now he was gone. Forever.

I still had three kids to look after. I soon recognized that I would have to lead them through this. If I came through this okay, they would be okay. But we had all been traumatized. Months went by and we started to resume a routine. A little emotional healing had taken place, which opened me up to a new phase: Anger. I began to feel the fury.

I explained it to my children. I said that I thought my anger was starting to come out, and I needed to focus it on someone or something before it took over. I didn't want to direct it toward my children, my friends, or people who didn't understand. My support system was obviously more important than ever. It was actually through harnessing these powerful emotions that I started to find meaning again. The first step was joining a support group with other Pan Am flight 103 families. We all shared the same experience and understood each other's feelings. We were going through the same grieving process. We didn't have to explain or defend our reactions. Through the process, I began to realize that Frank really wasn't alone that day. He was in the company of good people, with wonderful families back home. My mind was now stepping outside of my loss and was starting to register the bigger picture. This was the beginning of true healing for me.

The Pan Am flight 103 families became an extended community. Valuable friendships were formed that still endure today. And we began to apply what we had learned. A second milestone came on September 11, 2001.

I immediately started a support group for wives who lost husbands that day. I partnered with a dear friend who lost her husband on Pan Am flight 103. We hosted weekly support group meetings in our homes. We supported the widows emotionally and in every way we possibly could. My kids were more concerned about me going back in time, but to be honest, it helped me to help them. They would ask us things like, 'Does the pain ever go away?' We were very honest with them; we told them that it doesn't. But we explain how it changes. When this happens, you get a big hole in your stomach—that hole is the person you lost. That person is gone and you can never replace him. But what happens is that you shrink that hole in your stomach with little things the rest of your life. And it fills up again with a lot of little things.

When you see the expression of someone change because you have really connected with her, and helped her, it's a terrific feeling. So I was willing to do that over and over again. Five years later, I take great pride in seeing how they have progressed. They are further along than I was after five years. The key is that they had the proper support, right away.

Currently, I'm also in the process of initiating an ongoing program for Northern New Jersey on traumatic grief—surviving the loss of a loved one to a traumatic death. This program has been highly successful in the southern part of the state and so I held a fundraiser in my husband's memory to raise funds to bring it to northern New Jersey.

Today, I have five grandchildren, I have two great sons-in-law, and my kids are doing well and living full, happy lives. I have many wonderful nieces and nephews. All these things are things my husband can't share with me, but I'm still glad to have them. These are the things that fill you up over the years.

When my husband first died, it was like I wanted to die too. But now I realize I would have missed out on all of this. I believe that I still have a long life ahead of me. I see my aunts and parents living well into their nineties and it's important to me, knowing that I have longevity on my side, to make my life have meaning."

Think about the things that you take notice of during the day—things that may even dismay you. What issues do you talk about with friends, family, and neighbors? For example, you may live in a part of the country that is very scenic and laid-back, and you may fear the encroachment of developers. By all means, get involved. This is not a time to roll over. The world has enough problems as it is, without people destroying its natural beauty. Fight. Get passionate.

You don't even have to start big. In this case, you could begin by organizing a cleanup day in your neighborhood. Get some neighbors together and just start picking up all the trash. Through this small chore, you will soon find yourself connecting with the earth. You'll see your world a little differently. A friend of mine did this with a group from her neighborhood one weekend. She watched a driver go speeding by and hit a deer. The deer died right at her feet. This particular region contains a

▶ **LIVING THE 100-YEAR LIFESTYLE:**
Jacob Plasker

"When my son Jacob was born, I was a proud papa. I had grand visions for his life and believed he was destined for greatness. I couldn't wait to share an incredible life with him. I believed he could live an extraordinary 100 years. And when he was born, he had everything in place to be able to do that. Unfortunately, when he was ten months old, he had an accident that caused him to be paralyzed. All the experts told us that he would never walk, talk, or use his right arm. And through a strong belief in the healing powers of the human body, incredible faith, and a lot of the self-care, health care, and crisis care strategies mentioned through the 100-Year Lifestyle, he has regained his potential. At 16 years old he has an incredible life ahead of him and he has grown into a dynamic, handsome, and quality young man. His healing inspired my passion for human potential to a whole new level. This power to heal, be healthy, live in abundance, and make a difference in the world is in every one of us. It is the essence of the 100-Year Lifestyle."

large nature preserve being consumed by developers. She told me that when she saw the impact, firsthand, it deepened her desire to preserve the region where she lives.

I recently chose to put a lot of energy into the nonprofit organization founded by Stedman Graham in 1985 called Athletes Against Drugs. This organization exists to inspire and educate kids on the importance of living healthy, drug-free lives. My kids are now teenagers and, obviously, I want to keep them safe, healthy, and drug free. I feel very strongly that there are too many young athletes using drugs—both performance enhancing and street drugs. They think it will help them compete, but they are not approaching this with their best 100-Year Lifestyle in mind. They are not thinking long-term and many are simply ignorant about the consequences of their choices. Connecting to this cause keeps my passion burning to make a difference in the world. It is exciting. I have gotten to meet great people who are involved in the organization. I have tapped into new avenues of creativity, and I feel a strong sense of purpose every day because of my commitment. If this cause sounds exciting to you, visit their Web site at *http://insightforyouth.com* and get involved.

There are so many ways to get involved and make a difference.

Being in service is one of the greatest gifts you can give to the world, and it is also the greatest gift you can give to yourself. Why wait until you are gone? If you are going to live longer than you ever thought you would, why not make it worthwhile? Give yourself permission to engage in your life in a way that you never have before.

Centenarian Secret If at any time in your life you've had a burn in your gut to do something, accomplish something, try something, and really express your heartfelt passions, now is the time to do it. The truth is, desire has probably always been with you and will never really go away. It may dim from some challenges in life. But just like a fire, if you give it a little poke, the flames reignite.

I want to live in a world where people everywhere are making their lives matter. I want my children and their children to experience a world where people are committed to creating meaningful legacies and living passionate lives. Anything is possible when you tap into the depths of your own human potential.

I truly believe that everyone deserves to be healthy and to express their full potential—from the time they are born through their last breath of life. The choices we make today will impact our quality of life today and in our future. They will also impact the world, since we are all more intimately connected than ever before. I want to live in a world where this is happening. I would love to experience the beauty of that world for myself, my family, and my future grandchildren, a world in which people are living their full potential—truly living their ideal 100-Year Lifestyle.

HERE'S TO US

I would like to end this book with a nod to my wife's grandfather, Hyman Sperling, who turned 100 on December 7, 2006. He and his wife, Henrietta, were married for 60 years. His advice, which has always stayed with me, is brilliant yet simple: "Be true to your loved ones, your friends, and your buddies. Closeness and companionship are all you need." I would like to add one more thing to that: Be true to yourself. Be true to your heart's desire and live with passion. Have you ever noticed that people who live with passion just seem to get better, year after year? That's what the 100-Year Lifestyle is all about: living an incredible life, every day of your life, for 100 years and beyond. So, here's to us. May we all enjoy and experience a sensational century. Meet you there. God bless.

THE 100-YEAR LIFESTYLE
ACTION PLAN FOR LASTING CHANGE

1. *Live your legacy every day.*
   Starting with today, make every interaction you have with other people a positive one. Look for the good in each person and stand for your best legacy today.

2. *Have gratitude for your past and look to the future with the promise
    of your ideal 100-Year Lifestyle.*
    What are the changes you know you need to make to live
    the legacy that resides in your genetic core? What would you
    like to see in your lifetime? Go for it. If you don't, you prob-
    ably won't see it. If you do, you surely will.

3. *Lead yourself.*
    Nobody is going to do it for you. You know what is right for
    you. Lead yourself.

4. *Develop your professional, community, and global leadership skills.*
    Get involved in your profession and continue to develop your
    skills. Set goals that will force you to learn the necessary
    skills you will need to live your ideal 100-Year Lifestyle.

5. *Get involved. Get active.*
    Choose a cause that matters to you and commit yourself to
    making a difference. Let your voice be heard.

6. *Embrace your family and multiple generations.*
    Look around you and identity both the younger and older
    people in your life that you would like to get to know better.
    Make a phone call. Get a date on the calendar.

7. *Enjoy a sensational century.*

I CHOOSE MY LIFE
By Dr. Eric Plasker

I choose to die.
I choose to live.
I choose to hate.
I choose to love.
I choose to close.
I choose to open.
I choose to cry.
I choose to laugh.
I choose to deny.
I choose to believe.
I choose to ignore.
I choose to hear.
I choose to be right.
I choose to relate.
I choose to scatter.
I choose to focus.
I choose to work.
I choose to play.
I choose to be angry.
I choose to accept.

I choose to despair.
I choose to hope.
I choose to give up.
I choose to persist.
I choose to suffer.
I choose to heal.
I choose to destroy.
I choose to create.
I choose to fail.
I choose to succeed.
I choose to extinguish.
I choose to ignite.
I choose to get by.
I choose to excel.
I choose to follow.
I choose to lead.
I choose to drift.
I choose to commit.
I choose my choices.
I choose my life.

APPENDIX
RESOURCES

For more information about keeping yourself healthy for the remainder of *your* 100 years, visit the following Web sites:

The 100-Year Lifestyle:
www.100yearlifestyle.com

Aerobics and Fitness Association of America (AFAA):
www.afaa.org

American Association of Retired Persons:
www.aarp.org

American Cancer Society:
www.cancer.org

American Chiropractic Association:
www.americhiro.org

American Council on Exercise:
www.acefitness.org

American Diabetes Association:
www.diabetes.org

American Foundation for Suicide Prevention:
www.afsp.orgdr

American Heart Association*:*
www.americanheart.org

American Lung Association:
www.lungusa.com

American Stroke Association:
www.strokeassociation.org

American Yoga Association:
www.americanyogaassociation.org

AOL Money & Finance:
http://money.aol.com

The Best Natural Health Information and Newsletter:
www.mercola.com

Environmental Protection Agency:
www.epa.gov

Federation of Straight Chiropractors and Organizations:
www.straightchiropractic.com

International Chiropractors Association:
www.chiropractic.org

International Fitness Professionals Association:
www.ifpa-fitness.com

International Sports Sciences Association:
www.issaonline.com

Massage Therapy Foundation:
www.massagetherapyfoundation.org

MSN Money:
www.moneycentral.msn.com

National Exercise & Sports Trainers Association:
www.nestacertified.com

National Association of Homebuilders:
www.mahbc.org/greenguidelines

Organic Consumers Association:
www.organicconsumers.org

Organic Trade Association:
www.ota.com

Spafinder: The Global Spa Resource:
www.spafinder.com

US Green Building Council:
www.usgbc.org

WebMD:
www.webmd.com

World Federation of Chiropractic
www.wfc.org

World Wide Online Mediation Center:
www.meditationcenter.com

Yahoo! Finance:
http://finance.yahoo.com

INDEX

▶ JOIN THE CLUB

The 100-Year
Lifestyle Club

Connect with the information, people,
and resources to help you live your Ideal
100-Year Lifestyle.

Visit **www.100yearlifestyle.com** today!

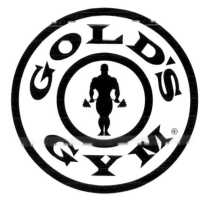

Change Your Body. Change Your Life.™

FREE One-week trial MEMBERSHIP

courtesy of Gold's Gym and *The 100-Year Lifestyle*™

800-99-GOLDS or visit Goldsgym.com
for the gym nearest you